Lulu's Secrets to Looking Good

Lulu's Secrets to Looking Good

Collins
An imprint of HarperCollins
HarperCollins Publishers
77–85 Fulham Palace Road
London W6 8JB

www.collins.co.uk

First published in 2010 by Collins

10 9 8 7 6 5 4 3 2

Text © Lulu 2010

Lulu asserts the moral right to be identified as the author of this work

Portrait photography © Paul Cox
Still-life photography © Noel Murphy
Exercise photography © Jerry Young
Stylist: Jillie Murphy
Commissioning Editor: Laura Kesner

A catalogue record for this book is available from the British Library

ISBN: 978-0-00-731054-8

Designed by 'OME DESIGN
Cover design by Heike Schüssler
Printed and bound in Frome, Somerset by Butler Tanner & Dennis

While every effort has been made to provide credits for the clothing and accessories that appear in the book, the publishers would like to apologize for any errors or omissions and will be pleased to amend credits accordingly in any future editions of this book.

Love this book? Visit www.BookArmy.com

Contents

Introduction

We are so lucky to be living at this point in time, which enables us (and encourages us) to look good for a lifetime. As a 15-year-old at the start of what has been a truly amazing career, I could never have imagined that I'd still be singing and performing more than 45 years later — and that strangers would stop me all the time to ask what my 'secrets' are...

'...WHEN WE LONG FOR LIFE WITHOUT DIFFICULTIES, REMIND US THAT OAKS GROW STRONG IN CONTRARY WINDS AND DIAMONDS ARE MADE UNDER PRESSURE.'

Peter Marshall

I wouldn't go back to being that 15-year-old again for anything. I am so much happier with my life now. I like to think that I have a little wisdom — which comes with age. But over the years, I have been incredibly lucky to work with some amazing professionals in the worlds of fashion, hair and make-up who have taught me how to make the very best of myself.

I've met a lot of women who think it's all over when they hit 40. I say: 'Forget about it, girl, because it doesn't even *START* till you're 40!' I know; I've been there. And I know that I'll be trying to look my best until I'm 80 and beyond, God willing!
I never go out looking like a bag lady and I even put on lipgloss to walk the dogs. I love glamour and I don't think there's enough of it around any more.

I'm not pretending that when you look at me you don't see a line, or any signs of ageing. I'm human, for heaven's sake. Up close you'd never think I'm a 30-year-old, or a 40-year-old — or even a 50-year-old — but I look as good as I possibly can for my age. It wouldn't be natural to look in the mirror at this age and not see

lines or shadows, but there's a lot you can do to fix that. It's all
about making the best of yourself. I certainly don't wake up in
the morning, look in the mirror and go, 'You gorgeous thing!'
But sometimes you put on the right outfit, your hair's looking just
right and your skin's glowing, and you think, 'You don't look bad
for an old girl!' So what I'm going to tell you in the following
pages is every single secret I've ever learned along the way.

The Very Beginning

My quest to make the best of myself all started when I was a
teenager. I believe I was destined to sing: at the age of five
or six I was already going to competitions which my mum and
dad would take me to. By age ten, I'd joined a concert band —
one of my uncles was looking for a female singer for his
accordion band — and every Sunday night I'd be singing on
stage. Then I was discovered by my personal manager Marion
Massey and, before I knew it, I was on *Juke Box Jury* and *Ready,
Steady, Go*, and working with people like The Beatles, The
Rolling Stones and Jimi Hendrix. Until that moment, I didn't pay
that much attention to what I looked like. Although I loved
clothes and was obsessed with hair, it was much more about
the singing and the music. But then I had to face the reality:
I'd never seen myself up close from every possible angle. I was
interviewed for magazines and newspapers and I had all these
images coming at me — and I didn't always like what I saw.

When I started out, I was probably typical of all the girls out there
— not everyone looked like Jean Shrimpton, that's for sure, and
I certainly didn't! I wasn't overweight, but I was curvier than
the supermodels of the day. My face was round as a football.
I wasn't tanned, or tall with long legs that went on forever, and I
had boobs, rather than the flat chests that were so fashionable at

the time (and as for the hair, it was back-combed up the wazoo!). It didn't seem to matter too much with my audience that I didn't fit the typical stereotype — girls wanted to dress like me and I even ended up with a ten-year contract with Freemans, the mail-order fashion catalogue — but it mattered to me.

I am very much my own critic, and I decided when I started seeing images of myself that I would work on my appearance. From that time onwards, I learned to be objective about myself, and turned to the best experts I could find in the worlds of hair, make-up, fashion and well-being in order to help improve myself. It's been fascinating, learning and watching what they've taught me. And through absorbing it all like a sponge, I've learned to accentuate the positive — and if I haven't exactly eliminated the negative, then at least I've tried to create enough distractions so you don't notice the bits I'm not quite so thrilled about!

Age is a State of Mind

But for me it's just as much about feeling great as it is about looking good. I am not about to put my feet up or go quietly into the sunset. I want to be able to dance, and sing with people who are younger than me, and travel and challenge myself constantly. Age is a state of mind nowadays, not a date in a passport. I think if you stay young at heart, that's half the battle. Not so long ago, I was working in California and three friends and I decided to go to Disneyland — no kids or grandchildren in tow, just us! Of course it's wonderful to take kids somewhere like that — but you don't need an excuse to do something spontaneous that gives you joy and brings you laughter. We had a blast, never stopped laughing hysterically from start to finish, while half-scaring ourselves to death on Thunder Mountain and Space Mountain. That Disneyland trip was something we did for our 'inner kids', and *that* keeps you young. I bought myself a pair of Tinkerbell PJs, which have become my absolute favourite pyjamas and, whenever I put them on, I remember that day, and how young and excited and happy we all felt, and it makes me smile like a seven-year-old. Was it 'age-appropriate'? We had a blast, so who cares? I am truly inspired by the people I see around me who are active and engaged with life at a much older age than I am. A friend told me recently about a video on the internet of a 70-year-old mono skiing — how great is that? Now, I'm not suggesting that you suddenly take up mono skiing at 70 — but how wonderful is it that she's kept going, and is still following her passion? She feels *alive*! How fabulous!

Your Inner Beauty

But I also truly believe that, as wonderful as skincare, make-up, haircare products, a great cut and the right clothes can be, you need to nurture beauty from within, too. That means eating the foods that will help your skin and boost your health — because that is the most precious gift of all, and one we need to cherish as we get older. It means finding a way of getting enough exercise to keep you fit, healthy and flexible, and that you enjoy while you're doing it. It's also about mindset, finding ways to calm down and cope with the crazy rollercoaster that is life in the 21st Century, with all its pressures and strains. If you're stressed, it shows on your face. A smile, by contrast, takes off ten years, like an instant facelift... Go figure.

I know that, like me, *you* want to look — and feel — your absolute best. And I also know that it can just go on getting better. So, let me tell you, I don't care if you're my age or younger — 50, 40, thirty-something, whatever. I've been there. I've done the work. I've picked up secrets from the best in the world. And all I can say now is: keep reading...

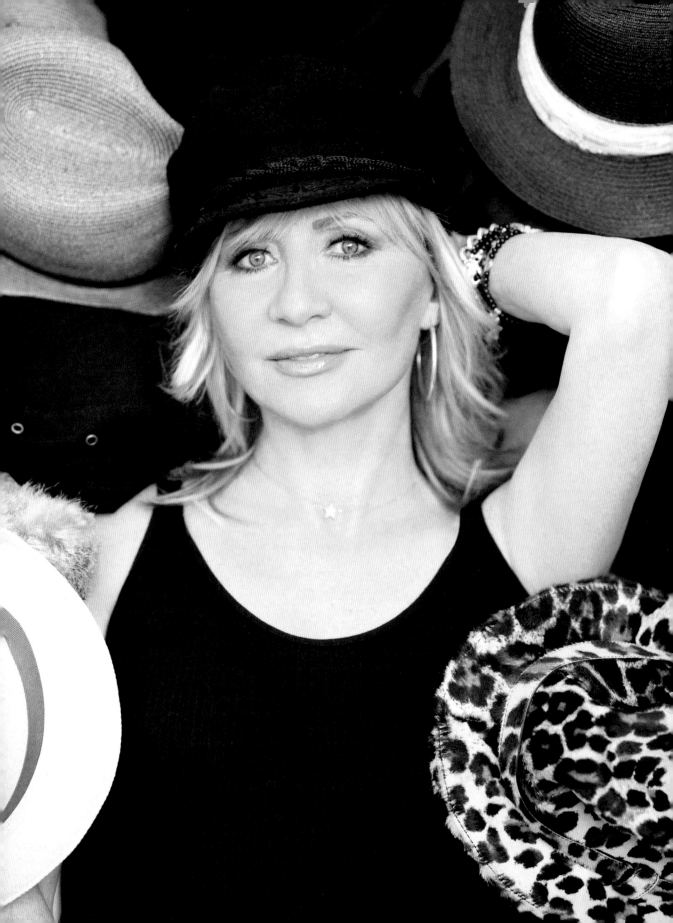

Skincare Secrets

Good Skin
Confidence

Today, in every way, I feel comfortable in my own skin. But, trust me, it wasn't always like that. And what I know now is that if *I* can feel good about myself, and my skin, then any woman can.

Of course, my skin has changed since I was a teenager — thank heavens! But those early skin troubles really zapped my confidence, and made me realise that how you feel about your skin is absolutely bound up with how you feel about the world. And how you *think* the world feels about you... Good skin = confidence. Simple as that. And, happily, there are plenty of secrets I've learned which ensure that my skin looks the best it can...

When I was first working in the music industry, I was surrounded by absolutely gorgeous, peach-skinned girls whose complexions were a world away from mine. Actresses like Judy Geeson, Britt Ekland and, above all, Patti Boyd. Patti was a true goddess, absolutely stunning. She was dewy and perfect — almost like a peach waiting to be plucked, if that doesn't sound too weird. I felt tremendous pressure to live up to that standard. They were golden and sun-kissed. I was pale and freckly — like a true Scottish girl. In fact, my skin was so white that my auntie Janey — my manager Marion's mother — used to creep into my room at night, when I was living with them, and stare at me because she couldn't believe how pale my skin was.

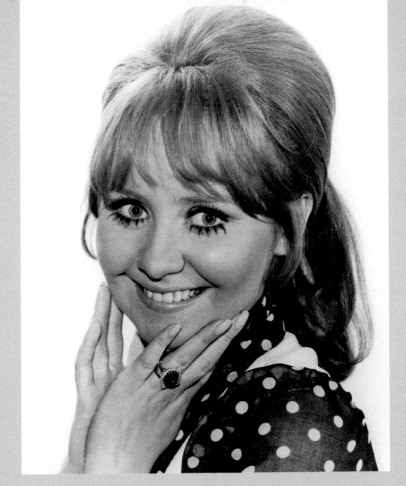

She used to say, 'You're so white, you look like you're from another planet!' But you know what? Being so fair has really helped my skin over the years, because I couldn't just slather on the Bergasol and lie out in the sun frying like so many of my friends with darker complexions did.

It's ironic now — because, like most women of 'a certain age', my skin is now dry, but as a teenager, I had the oiliest skin. Which meant that whenever I did TV or had my photo taken, they'd slap on the thickest PanStick make-up and dust me repeatedly with powder, just to keep the shine at bay. And because my pores were blocked with all that gunk, I'd get spots. My salvation came in the form of a wonderful Hungarian facialist called Countess Csasky, who was a well-kept secret among beautiful London women. A friend told me about her, and she began to transform my less-than-fabulous skin with her magic hands and the products and tips she shared with me.

Are you **ready?**

Wash *Away* Time

I had to learn how to cleanse my skin properly, because early on in my career it would literally be caked in TV make-up by the end of the day, and if I didn't cleanse, my skin would break out. Happily, my spotty days are behind me, but what I've learned is that, really, the most important thing you can do for your skin is to cleanse, cleanse, cleanse. Because, you know what? With skincare, if you aren't going to put in the work, you aren't going to get the results.

When I was younger, it was all about drying out my skin — so I even used soap, as well as an anti-bacterial cleanser that Countess Csasky introduced me to called Phiso-derm, which came in a distinctive green squeezy bottle. (She also used to dilute hydrogen peroxide with water and decant it into a little bottle that I travelled with, to pat onto my spots to dry them out.) But for anyone who's no longer a teenager, a cleanser absolutely *mustn't* over-strip the skin.

'IT TAKES A LONG TIME TO BECOME YOUNG.'

Pablo Picasso

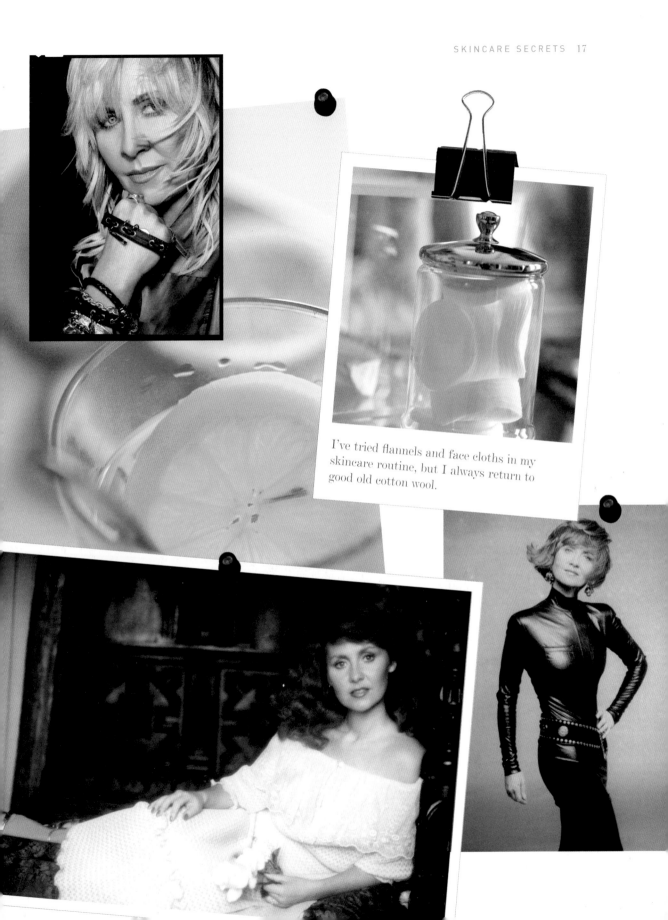

I've tried flannels and face cloths in my skincare routine, but I always return to good old cotton wool.

The right cleanser does the job in less than a minute, so nobody has an excuse not to cleanse — and there's absolutely no excuse to fall into bed with your make-up on. Find something that does the job. It's great if you love the texture and fragrance of your cleanser (or the fact that it has no fragrance at all), but frankly, I don't care if you use soap and water (if you even want to use facial wipes, that's fine, too — although I've never liked them because they leave a residue on my skin). But with cleansers, it's really a case of *just do it*! Slap your product on. Massage it in a bit. Take it off. It's that easy. And it can be that fast.

Personally, though, I like to take cleansing one stage further: I've found that having tiny, micro particles of magnesium crystals in my cleanser makes a huge difference to its effectiveness, literally lifting off the dead cells, revealing new, fresh, dewy skin underneath. So they're a key ingredient in my own cleanser, Take-Off Time Cleansing Cream. I'm obsessive about getting rid of those dead cells. It's all about regeneration — because fresh skin looks younger — and I can't emphasise enough how important getting rid of that drab outer layer is. (I'm so obsessed you're going to read about it again on the next page!)

I know women who don't believe in moving the skin on their faces around at all because they're worried that handling it too much will actually give them lines and wrinkles. But my experience is the opposite: massaging skin is just about the biggest favour that you can do for it. Massage gets the circulation going, and the improved blood flow does two things: it gives you instant radiance (and, beyond a certain age, it's *all* about radiance), and delivers vital nutrients to the skin.

If you can give it the time, one of the best windows most of us get for massaging our skin is when cleansing, working that product into the complexion so that it binds with any make-up,

BEAUTY FLASH...

Wash your hands with soap before cleansing, so you're not transferring germs to your face as you cleanse. I'm aware that I touch my face with my hands too often during the day — I can't help being expressive — but it's a terribly bad habit I'm trying to break.

cellular build-up (those flaky bits, especially around the nose and the cleft of the chin) and the grime of daily modern living. My tip is always to massage the product upwards, because that really works the cleanser into the pores. (And don't forget the neck and even the chest, which are so easy to overlook. Get right down there beyond the vest-line!)

Then you have to swoosh it all away. I've used hot towels, and big flannels, and then returned to good old cotton wool because I found that, when I was travelling, the flannels wouldn't dry out properly, bacteria would build up and they'd get manky, frankly. When I was creating my Lulu's Time Bomb skincare line, I wanted something even more efficient, so we came up with gentle skin-polishing pads to use in tandem with my cleanser: the buffing action makes the cleanser even more effective and helps with exfoliation — which I'm obsessed about, as you're about to discover…

I do love the feeling of water on my face: I start the day, every day, by splashing water on my face to wake up my skin — and wake me up, too. But in the evening, water can be part of a kind of ritual cleansing at the end of the day that can clear the mind before you go to bed, preparing you for sleep. I've found that it can be really helpful to literally imagine the stresses of the day, and any negativity, disappearing down the plughole with the water you've washed your face with. Bye, bye. Night, night!

I don't use toner. It's really not necessary, if you cleanse thoroughly (so don't listen to what the beauty consultants tell you!). If ever I feel the need for a little extra freshening action after my cleanser, I use good old rosewater, which isn't drying and just leaves the skin feeling fresh. Mostly, I don't even bother with that. My tip is to save your money — and your energy — and skip the toner.

Buff Stuff

One reason that skin generally starts to look older is that it begins looking drier and dustier and just doesn't have that youthful radiance any more. The reason, I've learned, is simple: cells turn over more slowly, and when they sit on the surface, they just don't bounce light back in the same way as dewy, fresh young skin once did.

This is why every woman of 40-plus needs to become a wee bit of a scrubber. In other words, exfoliate, exfoliate, exfoliate! I'm not talking about cosmetic peels or the kind of dermabrasion that you go to a cosmetic dermatologist's surgery for: those can be harsh and require quite considerable recovery time. I'm talking about daily skin-buffing to slough away those dead (and dead-looking) cells, revealing the fresh and more glowing skin beneath. Trust me: this daily microdermabrasion can be your fastest track to great skin.

Now I have my own skincare line, Lulu's Time Bomb — and these days that signature range is all you'll find on my bathroom shelf because the formulator (we call him 'Genius Joe') and I worked to create the exact products I'd spent so long searching for. So, as I say, the cleanser that I talked about earlier actually contains teensy particles of magnesium oxide, a mineral, to gently buff skin while it's melting away make-up. The key, whatever brand you use, is to choose an exfoliator with *gentle* particles — because your skin still needs to be babied, even while you're scrubbing it. Avoid harsh exfoliators with crushed nuts or olive stones, for instance, because the skin-sloughing particles have such sharp edges that they can actually scratch the skin and leave it red and sore.

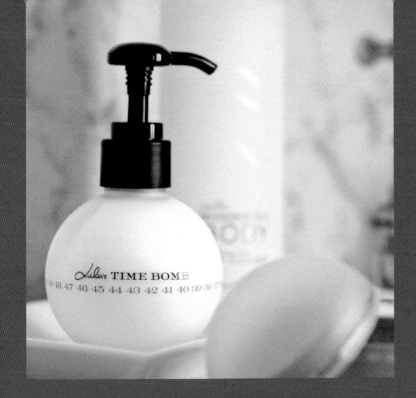

I stick to my own Time Bomb range now as the formulas are just perfect for my skin.

You can test an exfoliating skin scrub on the back of your hand, massaging it in using circular movements. If it feels too abrasive there, forget it, because it'll ultimately leave your skin feeling sore. What you're really looking for is something that's gentle enough to use every single day, rather than in a weekly blitz, because that's the way you'll see real, ongoing results. When I started daily exfoliation, I noticed that all of a sudden my skin started to look more regenerated, and brighter. As I say, this skin-buffing doesn't have to be harsh. If I can get away with daily microdermabrasion on the most delicate Scottish skin, then anyone can.

The trick is to massage your daily gentle scrub into wet skin, using those light, circular movements. So, if you can find a cleanser that combines sweeping away make-up with skin-sloughing, that's just perfect, because it will be working double-duty. Work it into the areas where skin cells build up, and avoid the eye zone, where the skin's thinner. By removing the dead cells, your skin's 'prepped' for the next step: your moisturiser or anti-ageing cream. And trust me, if you don't get rid of the dead cells, you might as well be applying that cream to old leather, for all the good it'll do!

Skin's
Glory Days

As I say, one big difference between young skin and older skin is the way light 'bounces' off it. In the 21st Century we get help on that front from light-reflecting particles found in many skincare and make-up products, which can create the optical illusion that skin is still in its glory days.

When you apply just about any moisturiser, it quenches skin, giving it that lovely, plump dewiness we're all after. The results, though, can be short-lived. So the best creams I've ever tried also feature light-reflecting mineral pigments, which literally bounce light off the skin. Not in a glittery way. Not even in an obviously shimmery way. But nonetheless, in my experience the creams that turn the clock back most effectively all have a little bit of gleam in them.

When I was younger, I never would have believed that my skin would one day become dry! Who can, as a shiny-faced teenager? But for most of us it starts to happen around 35 or 40 — and, before you know it, your skin's like the Sahara. When it comes to moisture, nowadays I find *more* is more — but I always religiously pat my skin dry before applying any cream, otherwise it just dilutes the cream's power.

Faces age in one of two ways, I've found. They either 'crumple' and become like crêpe — which is what my fair skin has a tendency to do (as do most paler skins) — or they develop folds and lines, which tend to be the result of excessive sun exposure,

To keep my skin looking dewy, I moisturise, moisturise and moisturise some more with a cream containing light-reflecting pigments.

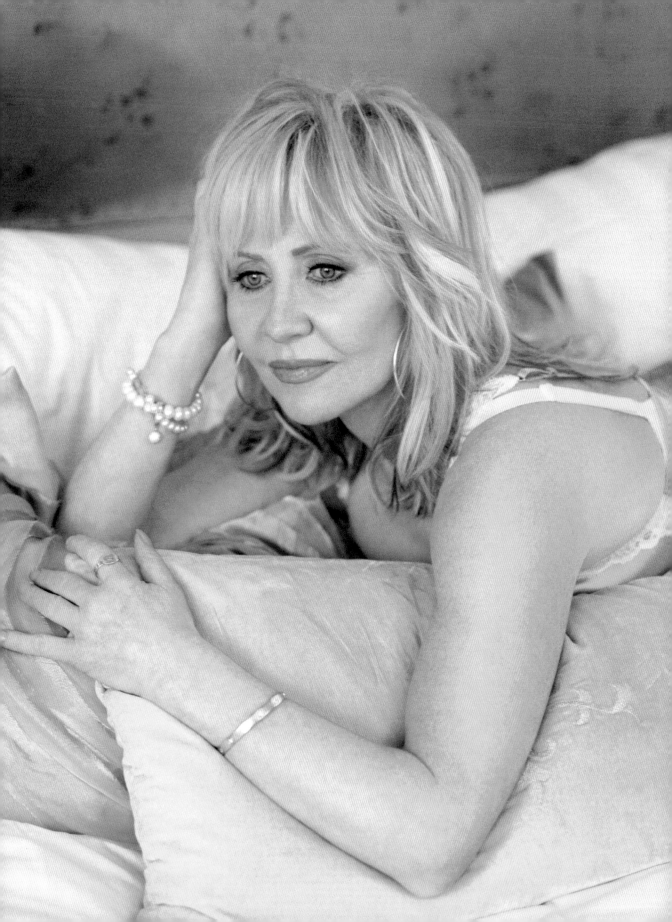

and a good reason to avoid the sun on your face at any age.
I believe there's a lot you can do from within to fight skin ageing
— including eating foods that are rich in antioxidants — but skin
creams can go a *l-o-n-g* way towards turning back the clock.
What *I* want in a skin cream is regeneration. I want all my cells
regenerated — inside and out. And, today I honestly believe
that's possible if we eat the right foods, supply our bodies with
the right nutrients and use creams that help to feed and
regenerate the skin. The right skin programme combined with
the right products can make a huge difference.

There really *are* creams that do more than just create the
illusion of freshness and youth: they actually regenerate and
nourish and put back what the skin loses as we age. And, at the
same time, they make skin smoother and more velvety to the
touch. I know now (and wish I'd known sooner!), that you don't
have to spend a fortune on them.

'SKIN CREAMS CAN GO A L-O-N-G WAY
TOWARDS TURNING BACK THE CLOCK.'

Mix and Match

Don't believe anyone who tells you that you can't mix and match products. I'm living proof that you can! At the first sign of ageing, I started using every product I could find: serums, oils, creams — you name it. In the past, my secret was to buy lots of products, mix them up and start blending them together: a touch of this, a smear of that, to create a cream that was rich enough for my skin, but didn't leave it so slippery and greasy that I couldn't apply make-up over the top. I became known among my girlfriends as this mad chemist, mixing and matching myriad lotions and potions. Over the years, I tried everything. EVERYTHING! From La Prairie to Crème de la Mer (I never got on with that because you have to work so hard to massage it into the skin). In the end I only got my perfect cream when I worked with 'Genius Joe' — my brilliant chemist — to come up with something that was skin-plumping, but didn't leave my face greasy or wet, didn't take an age to sink in before I apply make-up — and actually helped my make-up to stay put. (So many of those 'investment creams' made my make-up slide right off my face as the day wore on...)

As I said, what I've found is that the most skin-flattering creams all have that little bit of glimmer in them. How can you tell? Well, if you're trying a cream in a department store, apply a little to the back of your hand. Almost all creams make skin look vibrant instantly, so you need to wait a minute or two to look at your hand again. If there's a touch of sheen and gleam that remains after the moisture's sunk in and it's dry to the touch, it'll deliver that longed-for glow to your skin. What's more, that youthful glow will radiate from your skin even if you apply foundation over the top...

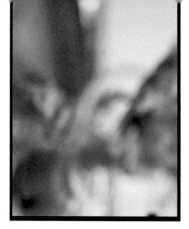

Youth Juices

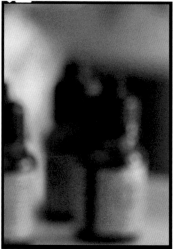

I first learned about facial oils and aromatherapy from Micheline Arcier, a true pioneer who brought aromatherapy to this country from France. It was absolutely new here when I tried it, and Micheline Arcier's name was also in the Little Black Books of many beautiful women. I learned from her the importance of massaging the face to boost radiance and which oils are the greatest skin-nourishers. She used to make up special blends for me and my complexion, which was making the transition from oily and breakout-prone to dry, which happens to most of us. I used to beg Madame Arcier to tell me where she got her oils, but she wouldn't tell a soul.

When I was in my thirties, I read an article about borage oil — and bought some in a health food shop. Borage-oil capsules can be a great introduction to facial oils: you simply break one open and massage it into the skin, and the essential fatty acids start to work their magic. (They're not called 'essential' for nothing!) At another stage in my life, I was simply massaging olive oil into my skin, and I also read that avocado oil works wonders — so I had a go with that. Believe me, I experimented with everything — but I found that those oils, used on their own, were too thick and greasy, and I hated the sticky feeling of having them on my skin because it gave me the sensation that it just couldn't breathe.

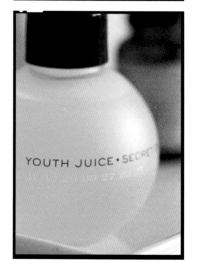

'THEY'RE NOT CALLED "ESSENTIAL" FOR NOTHING!'

What I've since discovered is that oils can be light (there are even oils suitable for oily skins, like grapeseed oil). They can sink in fast. And I've also realised that, actually, a more complex blend — specially formulated for faces — is much more effective than using something you might pour on a salad. The miraculous thing about aromatherapy essential oils (which you'll find in most pre-blended facial oils) is that they have 'synergistic' effects: individual oils boost the action of the others, which turbo-charges their magic powers.

One of the reasons skin becomes drier as we age is that its 'barrier' — which keeps moisture in — isn't so strong, because the surface isn't so smooth. This allows gaps to open up between the cells, allowing that moisture to escape. But you can use oils to help trap that precious moisture in the skin. So my trick is to 'layer' on cream over my oil. Honestly, I can almost *hear* my skin inhaling that facial oil! I slosh it on! I apply it to my fingertips, massage into the skin and give it a minute or two to sink right in. Then I apply my Flashback Night Cream over the top (or, in the daytime, I use Glory Days Day Cream. And yes, I *do* use oil in the morning — and I'll even run upstairs sometimes and put on a few drops during the day). And that 'layering' is what keeps my skin looking plumped-up and juicy.

Defy Time – and Gravity…

Up, up, up! That's the secret with applying facial oils and creams. I sweep oils and moisturisers upwards with my fingertips, in long, sweeping movements upwards from the neck, which ensures that every molecule of nourishment or moisture gets into the pores. (It's the opposite of the technique for applying make-up, which you can read about on p.66. If you apply foundation in an upward direction, it makes pores visible!)

Age-Defying Essential Oils

Frankincense — once used in mummification (and anything which can keep skin intact for 3,000 years must have miraculous powers!).

Rosemary — has a stimulating effect on the microcirculation of the skin, to promote radiance.

Chamomile — wonderfully skin-calming, with anti-inflammatory powers.

And these are also good...

Neroli — speeds up cell renewal, and is good for the treatment of stretch marks and scars.

Rose otto — especially good for skins (like mine) which are prone to high colour, as it strengthens capillaries and can even help to ease rosacea, which affects so many women nowadays.

Lavender — one of my favourite essential oils, partly because it's so soothing and calming to the senses, but also a great 'first-aid' fix for bites, bruises and burns.

Geranium — helps brighten dull skin.

The Ultimate Skin-Nourishers

Look for facial oils that include some or all of the following in the base. They're pure skin goodness, and packed with complexion-saving antioxidant vitamins that also work to reverse the damage done by pollution and sunlight...

Avocado oil

Olive oil

Sweet almond oil

Macadamia nut oil

Kukui seed oil

Sesame seed oil

A touch of my Youth Juice Serum smoothed upwards onto my face just before applying day or night cream locks in much-needed moisture.

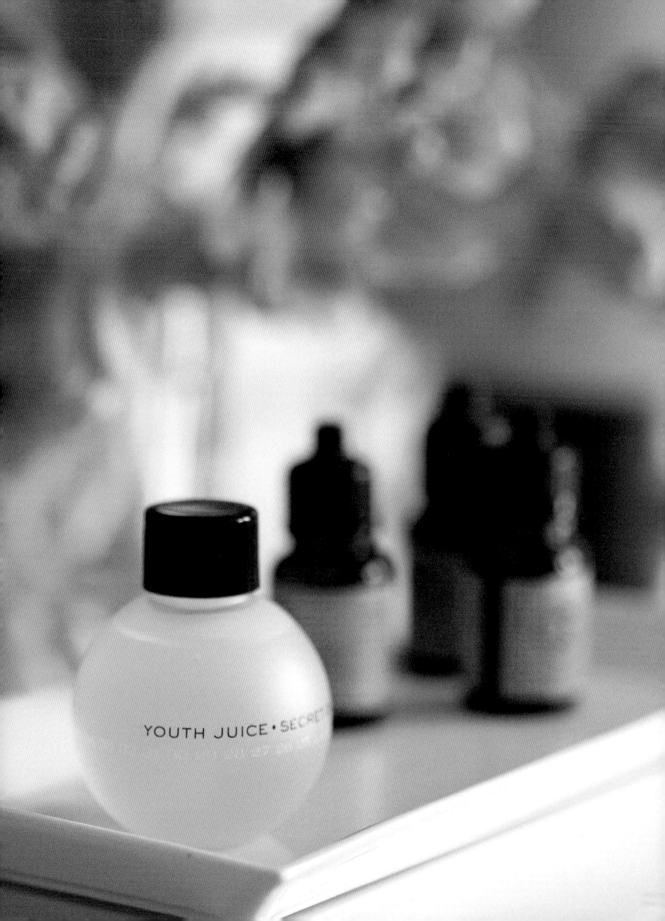

Smart Balms

From talking to friends — and all sorts of women, actually — I know that it's the lines around the eyes that bother them the most. Again, light-reflecting ingredients in an eye cream can do a lot to 'blur' the appearance of those lines, creating a sort of 'halo' effect that refracts the light so it bounces off the skin in a super-flattering way. So use the same trick when you're trying out an eye cream as a day cream: let it sink in. Then see if there's any residual gleam on the skin afterwards — in which case that cream's going to be good news for magic-ing away the appearance of those lines and wrinkles.

As the day wears on, though, that subtle sheen can disappear, with the result that the eye zone can look dry, and lines become more visible. That's ageing. So what I do is carry my eye cream around with me and use a dab or two during the day, even over make-up. I'm keeping the anti-ageing ingredients topped up, at optimum levels, but I'm also adding back that vital radiance, literally turning the clock back in the second or two it takes to pat my cream on.

The other bugbear women have about their eyes is puffiness — and sometimes dark circles (or, occasionally, both!). When I was working on my skincare line, my brief was really simple: NO PUFFINESS! I didn't want to wake up with any excess under-eye baggage. What I've found out is that, sometimes,

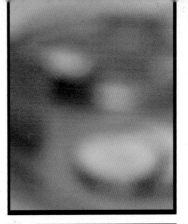

eyes are sensitive to creams because the creams are applied too close to the eye itself: you only need to dot an eye cream onto the brow-bone, and the 'orbital' bone around the eye, for it to do its job. While you're sleeping, your natural eye movements make that cream travel to the lid, and the under-eye zone. If you apply a cream too close to the eye — or it's too rich — then it can travel into the eye itself, triggering irritation and sensitivity, and swelling the tissues around the eyes.

Quick Tricks

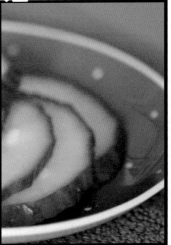

But if you *do* wake up with puffy eyes, I've got the answer: thin cucumber slices straight from the fridge and placed on the eyelids. If I wake up with a puffy face, I've even been known to put ice cubes in my basin, fill it with cold water and literally plunge my face into it! You have to be a bit careful with this if you're prone to broken capillaries, but if you stick to it once in a blue moon, it's an absolute miracle-worker — especially before a big event, or if you're about to have your photo taken.

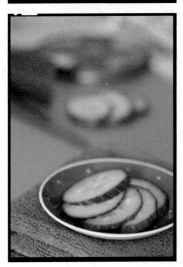

But you know what? When it comes to lines around the eyes, it's really worth remembering that when someone talks to you, they look *into* your eyes — not at the skin around them. Eyes really are the windows to our souls, and nobody I know — no man, or woman, let alone a child — is in reality going to look at you and see those lines. They'll see the sparkle *in* them. So when it comes to lines around the eyes, can I make a plea for a little self-acceptance? (As well as a dab or two of eye cream during the day...)

Try thin cucumber slices on your eyes for instant cooling and de-puffing benefits.

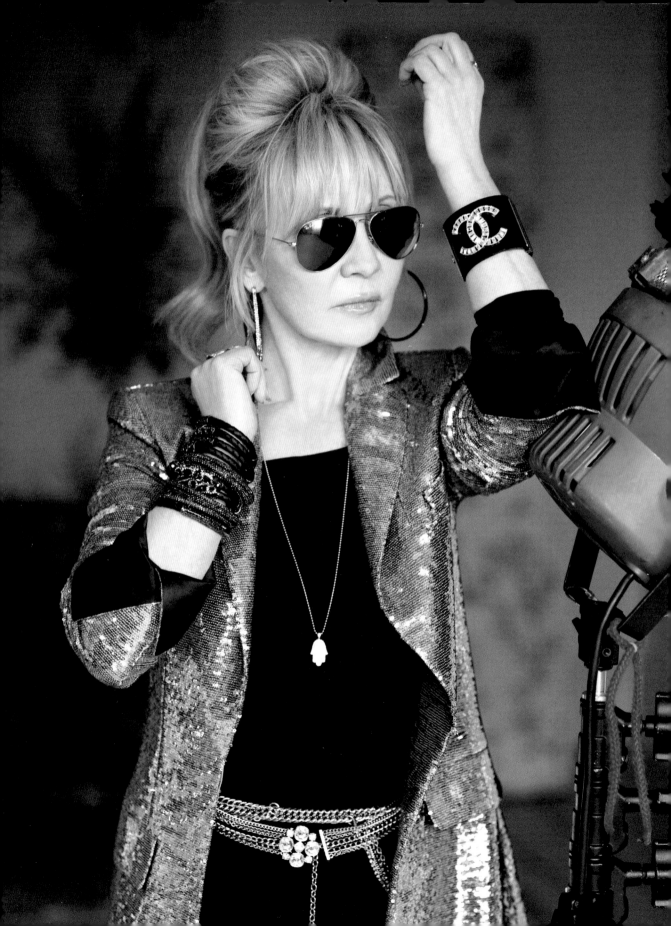

Stylish Sunglasses

There are two reasons the eye zone tends to develop lines before the rest of the face. First: eyes are more expressive — that's why they're so sexy — so the skin crinkles every time we laugh or smile. Second: the thinner skin is more vulnerable to sun damage, but it's also angled so that the sun strikes it more directly than the rest of the face. So I have a wardrobe of sunglasses that I wear outside, partly to stop my pale eyes squinting in bright sunlight, but also as a barrier between the skin around my eyes and the sun. When it comes to sunglasses, go for big lenses, dark tints and wide arms, if possible, which will keep the sun from damaging the skin at the side of the eyes.

'WHEN IT COMES TO SUNGLASSES, GO FOR BIG LENSES.'

Sunglasses add glamour to any outfit in a flash. The bigger the better for protecting the skin around your eyes.

Here Comes the Sun *(burn)*

Do you know how much I envied the gorgeous bronzed girls I was surrounded by when I first came to London? Imagine, this little, freckled Scots girl, down from rainy Glasgow, to find herself surrounded by beauties as sun-kissed and glamorous as Brigitte Bardot. I'd go on holiday with my new friends, who'd lie out in the sun going this gorgeous toasted colour. So I'd try to sunbathe, and I couldn't do it — because I'd literally just go beetroot. In those days, you didn't put on sun cream to protect you: you put on sun cream to *accelerate* the tanning (or in my case, burning!) process. I remember being on honeymoon with Maurice Gibb, and I woke up pink from top to toe, with this red hair — and Maurice and his brother Barry (and Barry's wife Linda) were this beautiful shade of bronze! Everyone else was splashing about in the water and I'd have to make a dash from under my umbrella into the pool, and back again into the shade. I was plagued by heat bumps and itching and it *really* didn't seem fair!

But, actually, it was a kind of gift. I'm truly grateful now that I didn't tan easily, because that spared me a whole load of sun damage. I'm still covered in freckles — the legacy of trying to tan, and if I stay out in the sun for any length of time, I develop more and more of them. But I learned to be religious about using sun protection, when sun protection factors first hit the market. And since then, I've never ventured out without being properly covered up.

I used to love the sun, but not what it did to my skin. Now I don't leave the house without my sun protection.

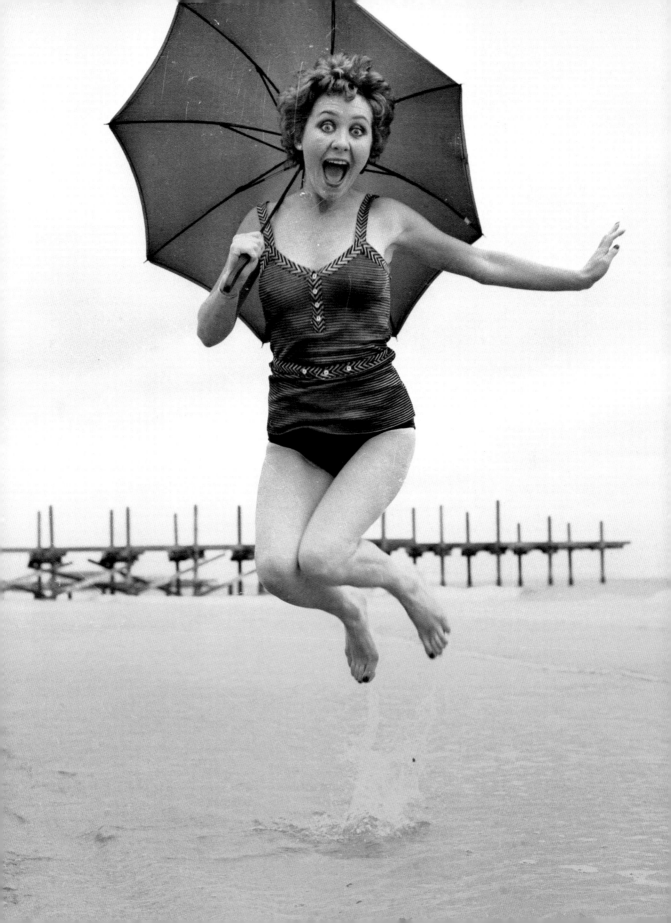

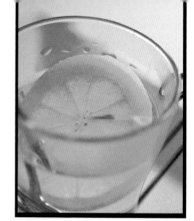

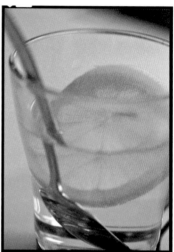

Facial *to* Facial

I learned a load about how to care for my complexion from my amazing skin guru, Countess Csasky. And what seems like a lifetime ago, *Vogue* published an occasional supplement called *Beauty, Health & Slimming* and I'd devour it hungrily when it came out. I learned so much from that magazine — I read skincare tips, and about yoga, and about places to go to get a facial, with names dropped by the great beauties featured in those pages, models like Ingrid Boulting and Jean Shrimpton, and actresses like the young Joanna Lumley. I realised very early on in my career that I didn't have the amazing physical gifts that models and so many actresses did, and so I was going to have to learn to make the most of myself. And it was the Countess — who was more the 'queen' of London facialists at that time — who taught me so much.

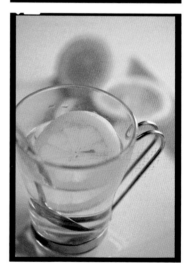

I was transfixed by her work, and by what she did to my face: her customisation of products for me is where I got the idea of doing it for myself. The Countess really did have healing hands, and it spoiled facials for me because I need to know that whoever is touching my skin *really* knows what she is doing. I'd arrive with my oily skin, which was always breaking out, and she'd get to work. She'd cleanse my face and apply hot towels to open the pores, and sometimes apply neat honey to my face, for its strong antibacterial effect — it worked wonders on my spots, though I hated the suffocating feeling! She would create a mask for my face using yoghurt, which I now know has lashings of lactic acid in it, delivering amazing, instant skin-brightening results. (I still sometimes do that, even now.) She'd add wheatgerm, and a touch of clay, and on would go the mask. By the time it was cleaned off, the mask had removed all the impurities and my skin was gorgeous (till travelling and the constant application of make-up for TV and stage shows clogged it all up again).

What that time on her treatment couch also taught me, though, is how important it is to take time for myself. And it's the same for every woman: unless you care for yourself, how can you start to care for the other people around you? Since Countess Csasky, I've been to see other facialists: Linda Meredith and Janet Filderman (and these days I occasionally see Arezoo, who's also a whiz at waxing) — but what I've learned is that it's *so* important to like and trust the person whose hands you're placing your face in. It sometimes helps if you can meet them beforehand, so you can literally check them out: do I feel a rapport with this person? And, personally, I'm always suspicious of those facials where they slather on 17 products and then give you an expensive 'shopping list' at the end of products you've just *got* to have for perfect skin. I want a facial, *not* a sales pitch!

Home Help

Instead of going for facials, these days I like to treat my skin to an occasional mask at home. I've tried them all, but long ago I gave up clay masks because they're drying for older skins. Now the masks I use are made of cloth, and infused with relaxing and skin-reviving ingredients. Soak the mask in a bowl of water, unfold and apply to the face (ensuring no bubbles are trapped and that the eye-holes and mouth-hole are strategically positioned!) and relax for 20–30 minutes in a hot bath (which, for me, is now a rare and special treat!). But I know that in a busy life, you haven't always got 20–30 minutes — so even 5 minutes makes a difference. Slow down. Breathe. Relax. Enjoy. And if you haven't got a face mask handy? Well, you've probably got a pot of yoghurt, so use a scoop of that, instead.

My Skincare *Adventure*

One day I was chatting on the phone to my very good friend Gail Federici, who used to run the global haircare business with my ex-husband John Frieda, helping to create products like Frizz-Ease and Sheer Blonde. I'd been complaining — not for the first time! — that in a magazine interview when I wanted to talk about my singing and songwriting, the journalist had given a lot of space to talking about the fact I looked good 'for my age'. So Gail said, 'You know, Lu, this is so blindingly obvious. Duh! If women all want to know what you put on your skin, why not create your own line, so they can do it too?'

Custom Blend

Up until then I'd custom-blend things myself because I figured that if two products were good, they'd be even better if I mixed them! I'd use a bit of this serum, a dollop of that anti-ageing cream and a swoosh of a special product that I used to get in LA from a man who made *only* eye creams. And then 'Project Shout' (it had to be!) was born. Gail reassembled the team who'd transformed John's range into a world-dominating haircare brand, who basically set about sourcing state-of-the-art ingredients, and responded to my shopping list for what I wanted for products for my fair, freckled, mature (God, I hate that word!) complexion.

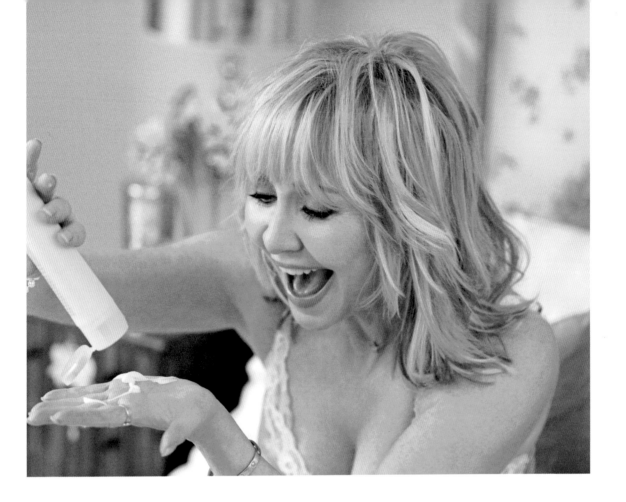

I turned into Little Miss Fussy. Many, many samples were FedExed back and forth until I was completely happy, and I became a human pinball going back and forth between London and the East Coast of America — which is one of the reasons why the whole process took three years. But, to be honest, the range has done so much for my skin that now I can get away without wearing a smidgen of foundation, a lot of the time. Without wanting to sound like an ad for my own range (though I hope I look like one!), if you turn to p. 264, you can find out where to get it.

But you know what? At the end of the day, it's all about finding products that you really, really, *really* enjoy using. Products which give pleasure to your senses as well as cleansing, moisturising and smoothing out those lines with dewy moisture and light-reflecting ingredients. Because products only *work* when you *use* them. Religiously. End of story.

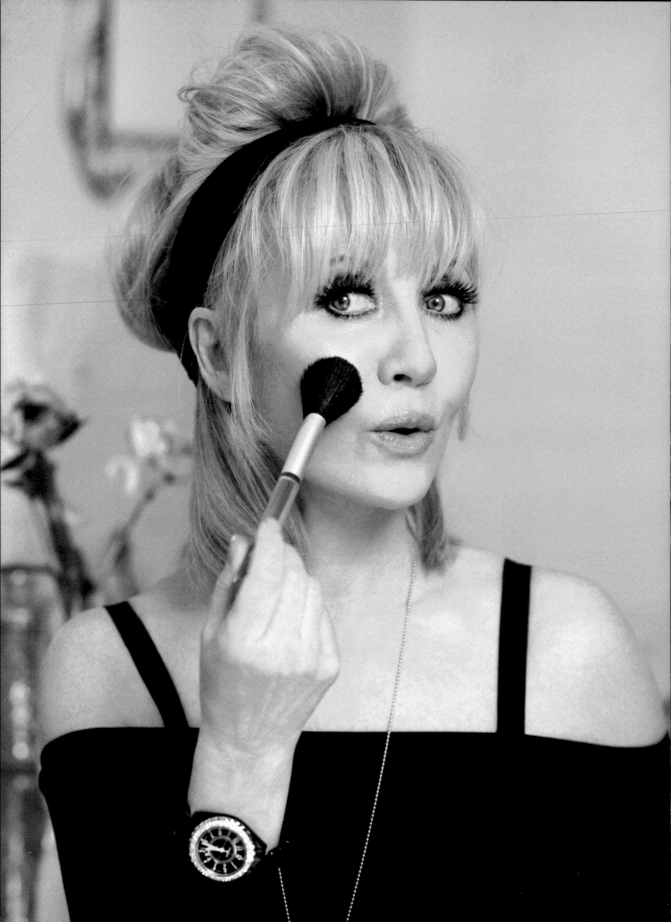

Making Up is *Not* Hard to Do...

Thank God for *Make-up*

And thank HEAVENS for the make-up we can buy now —
because it sure is a serious improvement on what I used to
apply, once upon a time...

Today, textures are sheer and gorgeous and make skin look
luminous. When I started out, textures looked like, well, a mask.
I wore PanCake and PanStick, which were created by Hollywood
make-up artists in the golden age of movies to cover absolutely
everything — so that you could barely see the skin! I figured if it
was good enough for the movie stars, it was good enough for
me, so I plastered on the stuff like it was going out of fashion
(which, happily it did, in the end...). Before that, I'd just copy my
mum. She had a bottle of foundation, and she'd do these two
stripes of lipstick on her cheeks like a Native American, and
blend them in as blusher. For my mother, lipstick was more like
a stain, so that's what I did, too. Then I'd add lots and lots of
mascara from a little compact that I used to have to spit in to
wet the brush! Happily, I've progressed a bit since then (and so
has mascara technology).

The whole point about today's make-up textures is that they
don't conceal everything: they just flatter your own complexion
so that you can get away with wearing the bare minimum.
Because, after 40, less really *is* more...

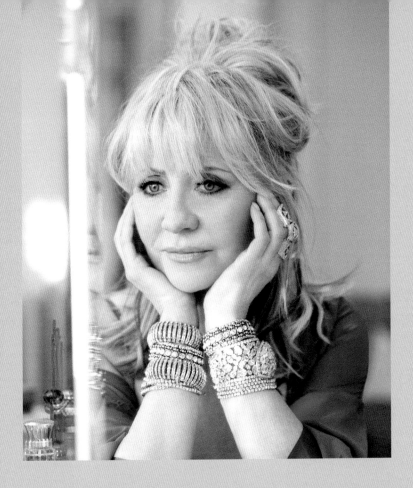

So for daytime, I keep it very simple. Of course for evenings — and especially for stagework — I go to town much more, as you'll see. (And, actually, stage and evening make-up can be pretty similar, because what you're trying to do is create that 'wow' factor from a distance.)

I'm lucky enough to have worked with some of the greatest make-up artists on the planet. I've had my make-up done by Barbara Daly (who became a good friend) in the early days, Mary Greenwell and — more recently — Charlotte Tilbury. I've also worked with the legendary American make-up artist Scott Barnes, who gave me the J-Lo look: He's literally like an artist, painting the face and using light and shade. It's a little scary to look in the mirror while it's happening, but at the end I looked *amazing*. Nowadays I work with a couple of make-up artists called Karina Woodruff and Gemma Smith-Edhouse. In fact, I've spent so long around make-up artists and models that now I know *all* the tricks.

Make-up brushes poised?

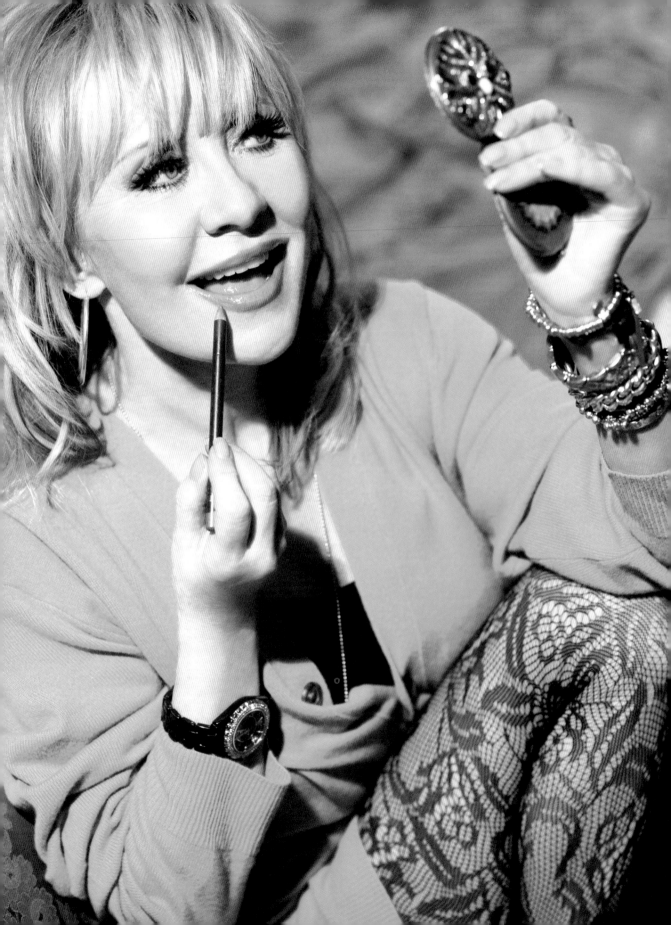

Light *and* Shade

Look at a painting of a face — the kind you might find in the National Gallery — and you'll see it's all about the contrast between light and shade. Well, that's basically what you and I are trying to achieve with make-up. These days we get a little extra help because, as I explained, a lot of make-up has those light-reflective pigments in the formula: those teensy little particles, almost invisible to the naked eye, but which bounce light off the skin.

Basically, make-up is all a trick of the light. If you learn to play with light to enhance your best features, you will look fabulous. It's that simple. So, after a certain age, you want to avoid flat, matte textures because they aren't youthful. You need a little gleam and shimmer and dewiness, because that's what looks young. Look at those old Hollywood movie stills, or a movie of Marlene Dietrich. She was so good at manipulating the light to bring out her best features — those cheekbones, those brows — that she was virtually her own lighting engineer. Once you start to understand how light works to enhance your face, you can become one, too.

Try this trick on your lips to see what I mean. Look in a mirror. Draw all over your lips with a lip pencil, or press on a touch of lipstick with your finger, so sheer it's like a stain. Then take a lipgloss and add a dab of it in the middle of the lip, and smack them together. Magic! Not only will your lips look instantly sexier, but youthfully plumper — and all because of a little trick of the light...

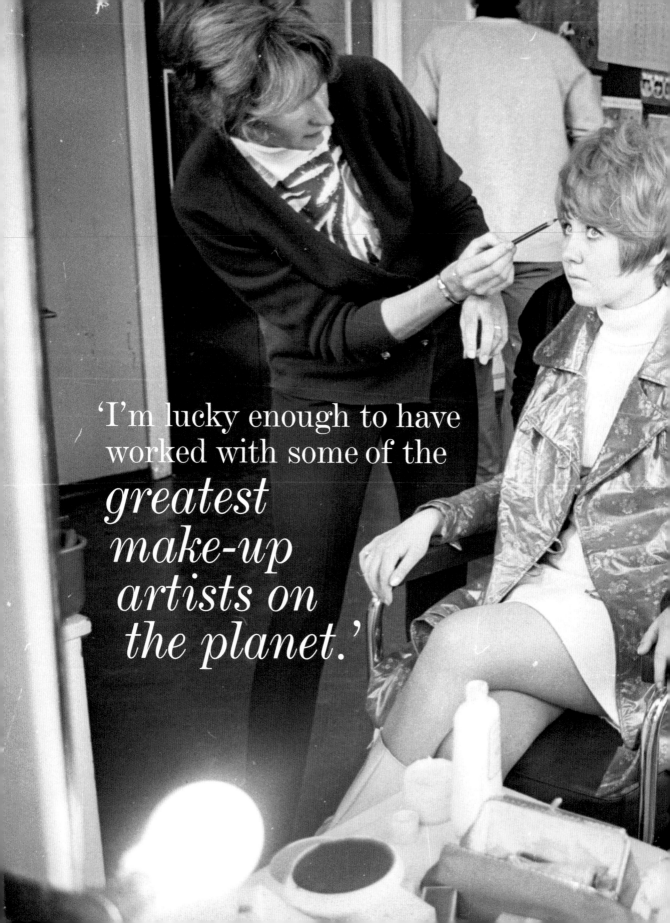

'I'm lucky enough to have worked with some of the *greatest make-up artists on the planet.*'

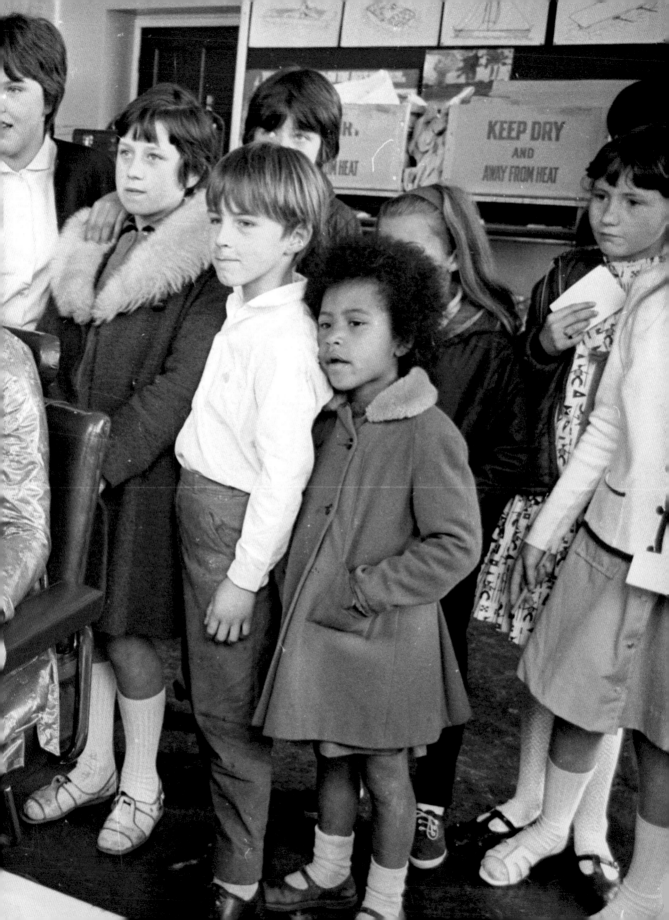

Prime Time

First things first: what really helps create the 'canvas' is to use a cream with light-reflective pigments as a 'primer' — to give skin a sort of candlelit glow. (I use my own Glory Days Cream, from my range, but for a tip on how to tell if a cream has those light-reflective pigments, turn to p.25.) And as for waiting 10 minutes for it all to sink in, a tip I read so often: honestly, I don't bother. I have all my kit around me; I just put on my Glory Days Day Cream, and immediately start applying my make-up. I do sit by a window to make the most of the natural light — always the best light to apply make-up in. If it's dark outside, I have lights around my mirror, but Barbara Daly says to take the shade off a table lamp; sit beside it and face the glow of the bulb.

Flawless Finish

As I said, I rarely wear foundation any more. (I promise you, since I started using my own Take Off Time Cleansing Cream, my skin tone is much more even and less prone to redness.) But concealer? Absolutely! After a certain age, I think concealer is *more* age-appropriate — because you don't end up with that 'mask' look. So after I've primed my skin with moisturiser, I reach for my light-reflecting concealer pen — which happens to be Dior Skinflash. (I used to be a Touche Éclat girl but I found it too drying and too pinkish in colour.) I pump it a few times to get the cream concealer onto the brush, and then I start drawing. Literally. I stroke the brush along the grooves that run from my nose to my mouth, and all around my mouth, too. (Then, when I put my lip pencil on, my lips really stand out.) I add a wee bit in the fold below my mouth, I blend with my fingers — and that's it.

I often apply a little eye cream over my make-up throughout the day to keep the thin skin moisturised and plumped up.

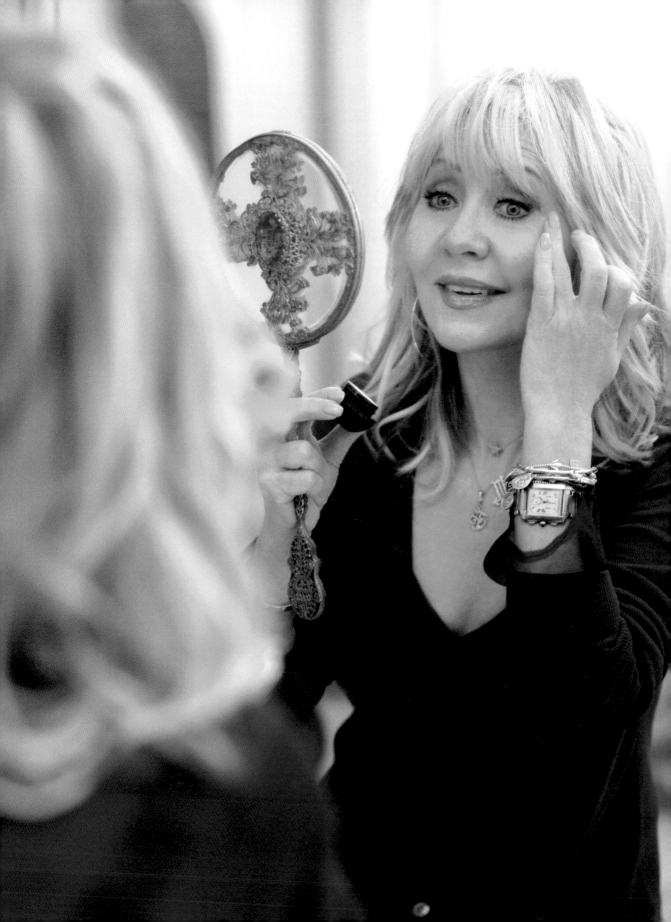

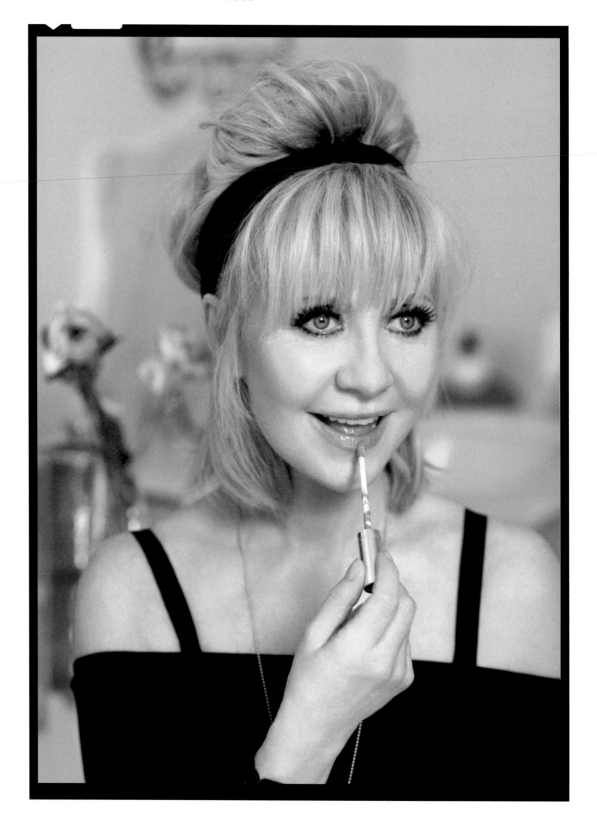

Lip *Tips*

Perfect Pencils

After I've used my concealer, my very next make-up step is to line my lips. One of the things I really notice is that most women I know don't bother with a lip pencil — but I can't live without mine. I have two, and they go everywhere with me. I even wear them on a 'dress-down' day, when I'm just walking my dogs in the park. They may be all the make-up I wear, with a pair of dark sunglasses to hide behind. Do without my lip pencils? No way!

Now, we're not talking about the kind of lipliner that gave lip pencils a bad name, way back — you know, the aubergine or bright red kind which meant that when your lipstick wore off you'd be left with a visible line all around your mouth. No, what you're looking for is a lipliner that's pretty much lip-coloured. (Although personally, I like to use two, to customise the perfect shade.)

I don't have a big mouth — but I do have a bigger one by the time I'm finished with my lip pencil! I basically draw all the way around my mouth — I even draw straight across the cupid's bow, to make my lips look fuller and less rosebudish. Yes, I go outside the natural contour of my lips, absolutely! And then I fill in with the pencil, just like a kid's colouring-in book. I know women who get their lips pumped up at the dermatologist's office so they look like a platypus — but why, when they can use a lip pencil and get a much better effect?!

Lining and colouring in my lips with a neutral pencil and then layering over a gloss keeps my pout looking natural, polished and kissable.

Look in the mirror and use the pencil to draw *outside* the natural lip line. Go on, try it! It's a miracle-worker. I start with my nude, slightly more peachy-beige shade of lipliner, which is MAC Subculture, and then I go over it again with MAC Dervish, which is a pinker shade. (I'm also loving MyFace Nude, on the outside, with Rosepetal all over my lips.) Together they make the perfect can't-tell-it-from-real lip shade.

Actually, those are shades that would work for pretty much anyone's skin tone, and they won't break the bank — but if you're buying from a high street range, go for the most liplike tones. No mahogany! No cherry! No way! And be sure to choose a super-soft texture — you don't want anything hard, or that's how the line will look when it's on your face. You're looking for something that smudges easily.

If you're trying a tester in a store, often they've been sharpened, so draw back and forth with it a few times on the back of your hand to get rid of the pointy 'tip' because that doesn't give you much of a clue. Draw on your hand again with the softly rounded end — and *then* see how soft or precise it is. Soft is good, but not *too* soft or it'll smudge. (In summer my lip liners get a bit *too* smudgey and so I keep them in the fridge.)

BEAUTY FLASH...

I mix and match make-up all the time — just like I always have with skincare, and with clothes. Just because there are four shades in an eyeshadow palette, don't stick to four! Blend them together in different combinations and see what you come up with. Mix two favourite lipsticks by smudging them together on the back of your hand, and see what colour you get. If you're feeling bored with the shades in your bag, you may not need to go make-up shopping: you can create a whole new palette with what you've got if you start playing.

Give it Gloss

I also occasionally like to apply a sweep of lip balm beforehand
to soften my lips. But it's important to blot it because it can
make the lip liner smudge. (I once accidentally put a little of my
eye balm on my lips and it worked a treat, so I've done it ever
since — and it's my secret for soft, sensual lips.) Or you can add
a little balm after you've applied your lip pencil, for a bit of sexy
glisten and gleam — just dot in the middle of the lips. My
favourite lip colours are MAC Viva Glam Lip Gloss and, if I want
something pale, MyFace Strawberry Fields, for a bit more
colour: it's sheer and glossy. If I want a peachy, pale gloss, I'll
go for MAC Lipglass in Prrr — which looks very modern.

Many women find that their lips become paler as they get older,
so this lipliner trick is a real godsend to enhance the pout. Me?
My face has got much paler, so my lips actually stand out *more*,
in contrast nowadays. But will you catch me out walking the dog
without my lipliner? *No way*, baby.

'BUT WILL YOU CATCH ME OUT WALKING
THE DOG WITHOUT MY LIPLINER?
NO WAY, BABY.'

Honestly, I've got it down to a science
... *So here's the step-by-step:*

1   A magnifying mirror is a must, especially if you need glasses. It's brutal, but worth it not to look like Bette Davis in *Whatever Happened to Baby Jane?* when you've finished.

2   I use a light-reflecting concealer (Dior Skinflash) all over the lid and on dark circles under the eyes (especially in the evening), which evens out skin tone (getting rid of redness or shadows), and acts as a 'base' for make-up to cling to.

3   I outline my eyes with a kohl pencil, close to the lashline — I have both black and brown Lancôme Le Crayon Kôhl pencils. (These are pretty impractical because they're really long pencils, so I actually break them in half to fit them in my go-anywhere kit!) Then I take a brush and blend the eyeliner pencil to create a softer line.

4   I don't like my brows too dark these days. I've been through phases of having them dyed almost brunette, but I think it looks softer to have them a few shades lighter. If I want to emphasise them, I use Dior Powder Eyebrow Pencil (in a taupe shade) and extend the outer corners — where my natural brows just disappear

5   Next, I move quite a distance from the mirror — because when I'm applying shadow I want to see the full impact rather than the finer detail. (When I'm done I just check in the magnifying mirror that it's all perfectly blended.)

6   I have a palette of neutral eyeshadows: coppery-gold, taupe, dark brown and a pale shimmering bone colour, and

I swirl quite a fat blender brush in the four shades to mix them. I then hold a mirror at a distance and use the brush to work the shadow mixture into my eye socket, spending time blending, blending and blending again, so that there are no hard edges. My palette is a customised quartet from MAC, with shades called Embark, Brown Down, Arena and Amber Lights. If you go to a MAC counter, they'll make up a similar palette for you, though, to be honest, I've got several palettes from other brands with pretty much the same selection of neutral shades; I end up buying them over and over. Basically, they are variations on the natural colours of the face and, in my experience, those are what work best for every woman. I have green-gold eyes, but I've seen these colours work beautifully on blue eyes and brown eyes, too, and palettes of those neutral browns are available for every budget. They're the 'Little Black Dress' of eyeshadow palettes.

7 I also use the brush to sweep the eyeshadow out towards the outer corner of my eyebrow. When I've enhanced the socket, I might also add a touch of the bone shadow to the brow bone, to emphasise the bone structure — and for that, I sometimes just dab it on with my finger.

8 When I've finished with the shadow, I reach for that kohl pencil again and outline the lines one more time.

9 I add lashings and lashings of mascara, till the lashes get really smoky. (My favourite mascaras — and I have road-tested them *all* — are DiorShow, and Maybelline Great Lash Mascara for a light day-time touch.) I wiggle the brush as close to the roots as possible. If I'm going on holiday I get my lashes dyed black so I don't have to bother with mascara.

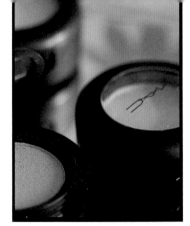

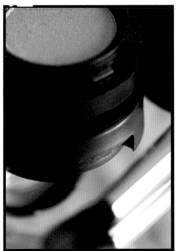

Smoky *Eyes,* *Glossy Lips*

I think that smoky eyes always look fabulous. End of story. The eyes really are the windows to the soul, and eye make-up is the window frame. I have a deep socket with lots of eyelid, so actually I can take a lot of shadow in the socket area, which is great for adding depth.

Magic Wand

When Dior discontinued the mascara with the best brush in the whole world — DiorShow — I simply rescued the brush, because it's perfect for combing through lashes to avoid any risk of that spidery look. (Simply wash a mascara wand in a little gentle wool wash liquid, sudsing it until it comes clean. Then leave it to dry on a towel, and keep it handy for use after applying mascara. You can do this with any favourite wand.)

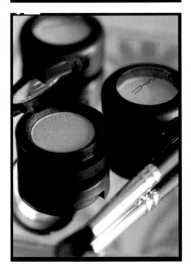

Colour Me Beautiful

Lipglosses are a bit like shoes: it's easy to be seduced into buying yet another one, and another one — and I've never met a woman who didn't love lipgloss. If you use my lip pencil trick, you won't need to use lipstick as well — but gloss, for me, is a must-have.

Again, it's really important not to stray too far from the natural colour of the lips. Sometimes I'll go a little paler, or choose a gloss with shimmering gold in it, but generally the shade is pretty close to my own natural lip tone. My favourite glosses are MyFace Mymix Lip Pop Lip Gloss in Fair (their shades are chosen to suit each skin tone), MAC Lipglass in Viva Glam VI (a pinkish-brown neutral, with shimmer) and Fran Wilson 0004 — not brown, not orange, not pink, but just gorgeous (with a touch of honey to condition lips).

Test for Texture

What puts a lot of women off lipgloss is the idea that it's going to be sticky, and your hair will somehow be magnetised to it. But believe me: not all glosses are created equal. If you're lipgloss-phobic, test the 'comfort factor' of glosses by trying them out in store — but avoid touching a wand to your own lips, for hygiene reasons. If you're shopping for gloss in a high street chain, take a little stash of cotton buds in your pocket to dip into the gloss and use to transfer the shiny shade to your lips (as well as a pocket mirror) so you can 'audition' it before you buy.

I apply lipgloss to both my top and bottom lips — and I've come to terms with the fact it's going to wear off during the day. But because of my lip liner 'base', I know that when it wears off I'll still have a lip-coloured pout underneath. And the great thing about gloss is that it's so easy to apply, you can redo it almost any time even without a mirror. Even in the back of a taxi with no lights on, if it comes to that.

Blush Stuff

How I used to hate my chubby cheeks when everyone around me — Patti Boyd, Julie Driscoll — had those fabulous sculpted cheekbones. But my mother was right when she said that one day I'd be grateful for them. Even now they're slightly plump and cushioned, which (at *this* age) is a good look. You can create that milkmaid plumpness and healthy glow with make-up, too.

Cream It On

I gave up on powder blusher years ago. After 40, cream blusher works best because it looks softer and blends better, with no risk of appearing dry and old ladyish. But the secret is to use a brush to apply it. My blusher brush is by MAC, and it's shaped like a fan (and made of synthetic bristles — essential for creamy and liquid textures). I touch the brush to the cream blush in the palette (usually Stila Convertible Colour; I use Lilium and Peony) — then I add a kiss, a whisper, a *breath* of blusher to my cheek: flick, flick, flick! It's always possible to layer on more blusher but if you try to take any away, you take everything else with it and have to start over (or risk looking like a panto dame all day).

Lots of women are confused about where to put blusher, so try this: take your blusher brush and imagine a line down from the centre of your eye — the pupil. Apply the blusher with your brush at the point where the line reaches the cheek. (The only women this trick doesn't work for, in my experience, is anyone who has naturally very ruddy cheeks, or rosacea. You want to keep any extra redness away from the cheeks, so apply your blusher further out along the cheekbones, towards the hairline.)

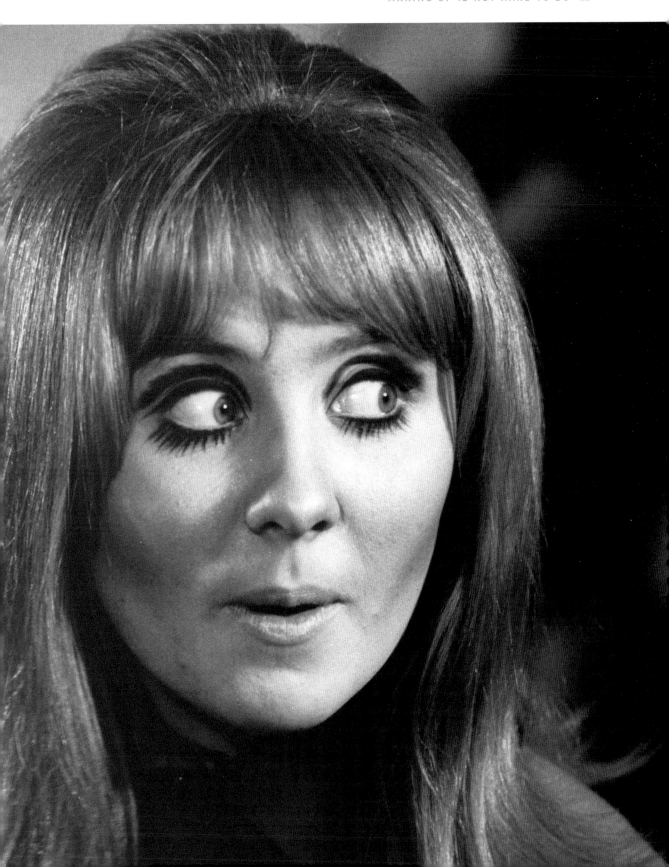

Perfect Powder

You do *not* want to look dry and dusty. But that's exactly how all-over powder makes skin look, and it is *very* ageing. Go for the very lightest, most translucent powder that you can find — it should literally be feather-light. Don't ever dip your powder brush directly into the powder, or you're bound to overdo it. There will always be a little dusting of powder in the lid of your compact or powder pot, so dip your brush in that instead. (I use Scott Barnes Translucent Powder, which is so super-fine that it feels like silk.)

The Best Brush

Traditionally, make-up artists use their biggest, fluffiest brushes for powder; I do the opposite. I have a small brush — no wider than two centimetres (about three-quarters of an inch) — and I use that to powder around my nose, and that's all. With a bigger brush, you can't help but get powder all over a much wider area, and you'll just look too matte. You don't want your nose to shine, of course, but everything else will look that bit younger if it's a little bit dewy.

'...EVERYTHING ELSE WILL LOOK THAT BIT YOUNGER IF IT'S A LITTLE BIT DEWY.'

Be a *Bag* Lady

How do you store your make-up? I like to see what's inside, to save time rummaging around looking for something. (File under: life's too short…) You can find see-through, zip-up bags in make-up stores, department stores or high street chemist's, in different sizes — they're everywhere now.

I have one kit that stays at home, and one for stage make-up that travels with me and a little Anya Hindmarch zip-up nylon bag, which isn't see-through, that I carry around in my handbag, with my absolute essentials. (You can see my list of must-haves on p.70.) You might also like to keep another in your office desk drawer or your sports bag…

The Nose Trick

This is not what you might think! It has to do with using light and shade, once again, to shape the nose. I apply light-reflecting concealer in a stripe all down the bone of my nose and blend. I then take a MAC Midtone Sepia Cream Colour Base — which is a contouring cream — and use my ring finger to dab a line either side of the nose bone, which I then blend. It makes my nose look longer and slimmer — and honestly, if you blend properly, nobody will be able to see that it's just an optical illusion. (I've heard Naomi Campbell does the same thing!)

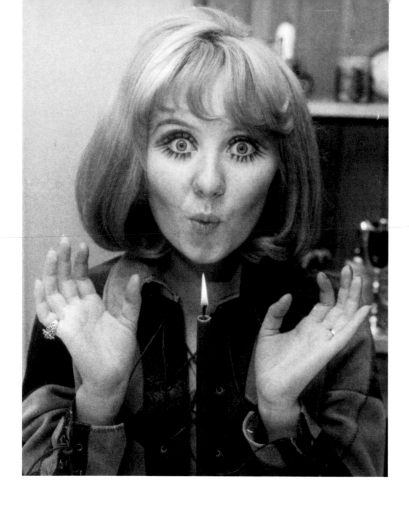

Makeover *Magic*

Maybe you've never had your make-up professionally done. Well, it's about time you did — because it needn't cost a penny. I'm very privileged: I've worked with some amazing make-up professionals, but there are talented make-up artists working in beauty halls up and down the country — particularly at the counters of big-name brands like MAC, Bobbi Brown and Chanel. It's a really good idea to book in, once or twice a year (or more often if you feel like it), for a free makeover. (Some of the counters take a small charge for makeovers — though most don't — but it's always redeemable if you buy something.) You will *definitely* pick up a few tricks, especially if you ask the make-up artist to let you have a go, too.

Learn from the Best

As they work their brushes over your face, keep looking in the mirror from time to time, so you can take in what they're doing. Let them do one eye and then try to copy it yourself using the same products and tools. Same for cheeks or foundation: they can do pretty much half the face and then you take over. (It's easier to remember how to do it yourself, when you get home, if you've had a go in the store.) Some make-up counters have special drawing pads pre-printed with the features and shape of a face, and the make-up artist can smudge on the products to create a 'blueprint', so that once you've left the store you can remember which shades go where. Once, when a make-up artist did my eyes, I had her draw a picture for me on a piece of paper. You think you'll be able to remember — but it's really hard.

I like having my make-up done by different make-up artists because it can be really helpful to have an objective eye assessing what might work for you — especially since lots of women get stuck in a make-up rut after a certain age. And the great thing about make-up is that if you absolutely hate the results, you can go straight home and sweep the whole thing off. But I bet you won't!

PS. If you really want to splash out, I can also recommend a make-up session with the wonderful Jenny Jordan, who did my make-up for shows and for photoshoots for years and years — until she opened her own Eyebrow and Make-up Studio and became too darned busy! Jenny's studio is in Belsize Park, London, and for more details go to www.jennyjordan.com. She'll go through your make-up kit, make recommendations and probably teach you a whole new way of doing your 'face', which will be a complete revelation — and will almost certainly inspire you to change the way you do your make-up forever...

Your Face,
My Face

It's really hard for someone who isn't a professional make-up artist to tell which colours will suit you when you're faced with a rainbow of shades at a make-up counter. My friend Gail Federici (my ex-husband John Frieda's business partner who helped him to create his haircare empire) had a brilliant idea a few years back, and got together with international make-up artist Charlotte Tilbury to create a range that takes all the guesswork out of choosing your perfect shades. It's cleverly divided into 'Fair', 'Medium' and 'Dark', and Charlotte chose the perfect shades within each skin tone to make them completely fool-proof.

Pick any product in your skin tone 'family' — lipstick, lip liner, blusher — and it's guaranteed to make the difference between drab and fab. (Charlotte says that once you get those basics right, you can experiment with eye colour and be quite daring. Although, personally, I'll be sticking with my neutrals, rather than the iridescent emerald greens or mermaid blues. Gorgeous shades, yes. But after 40, if you've got a passion for purple, I'd recommend indulging it with a cushion or pashmina, *not* an eyeshadow.)

I often go a bit darker with my eyes for evening make-up, but like to keep my lips and cheeks fairly neutral. Only play up one area of the face at a time.

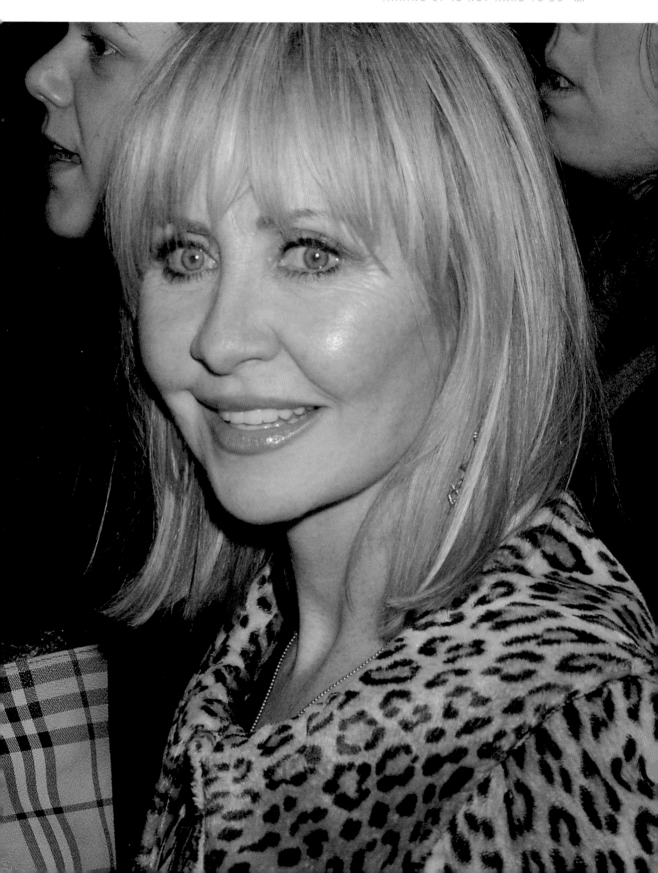

Lights, Camera, *Action*

The make-up I do for night-time, and for parties and dinners, really isn't that different from my everyday look: it's all about impact — and taking a little extra time...

✳ For after dark — and in front of the cameras — I use an amazing product from Terry de Gunzburg's By Terry range called Light Expert (my shade is No. 3 Honey Light), which is a super-sized concealer wand that dispenses gleaming concealer/primer all over the face. I blend with my fingers or a sponge, until it's seamlessly fused with my skin. But, you know I said that I always work my skincare products in an upwards direction to ensure they get into every pore? Well, it's the opposite with make-up: always apply in a *downwards* direction, to minimise the appearance of pores. If you press make-up upwards, it simply accentuates them.

✳ To create the canvas, I use concealer to make myself look pale in the t-zone of the face. I take my Skinflash pen and use it around my nose, around my lips — all the places I talk about on p.54, but especially around my lips so that when I put on my pencil, my lips jump out. OK, maybe not exactly like Mick Jagger's, but it's pretty darned effective.

✳ I give myself cheekbones by blending in Laura Mercier Tinted Moisturiser — what you get is a very realistic contour effect. I also sometimes use it just under my jawline, to sharpen up my jaw. You wouldn't want to do this every day, but for a photo or a special event, it's very face-slimming.

❋ I do my eyes using the same technique as on p.55, but even more dramatically. When it comes to smoky eyes, after dark, *more* is more.

❋ I curl my lashes then put on loads and loads of mascara, which I sweep through with my DiorShow 'rescued' mascara wand. Which curlers? Shu Uemura. You've probably read the name a hundred times in magazines, and there's a good reason: they've become a legend in the beauty industry because they fit the shape of the eye just so — and the rubber pads are ultra-gentle, so they don't tug or pull any lashes out. I use the double-squeeze method preferred by make-up artists: clamp the curler round the lashes, squeeze, let go and squeeze again.

❋ Sometimes, just sometimes, I'll go to town and wear false eyelashes. As a teenager I used to wear those big spiders, top and bottom, but now I go for individual false lashes.

❋ Last thing, I take a big fluffy brush and dip it in my MAC Bronzer (in Bronze — or Golden, if I'm going on stage). Then I look into the mirror and whisk the brush around the outside of my face — as if I was making an outline. It creates an amazing 'frame' for the features.

These are all tricks you can try at home. The key is not to try them for the first time when you're in a rush — they require a little practice. When you've got an evening to yourself, sit down with your mirror and your kit and play. See how you can use the power of light and shade to create a beautiful, sculpted face, and once you've got the knack, you can do it again and again.

It's All About The *Brushes*

Professionals wouldn't dream of making up a face without the right brushes, yet so many women still think they can get away with their fingers, or the teeny applicators that come free with products. But once you've got the right brushes, you'll realise that they absolutely, totally, 100 per cent make the difference to how long your make-up stays put (brushes 'work' the make-up into the skin) and to the seamlessness of the finish.

Opposite are the brushes I can't live without. It's important to use the right texture for the right job, too: natural bristles work best with powders, but for creams and liquids, use synthetic. If you try to use a natural hair brush with a liquid or cream, it just 'drinks' up the formulation, takes ages to dry out and gives a streaky finish. In my experience, the best brushes are by MAC. (Why do I keep mentioning them? Because their entire range is make-up-artist-quality. And that's what you're trying to become.)

Brush Care

As long as you give them plenty of TLC, good brushes will last a lifetime. I actually wash some of my brushes every single day — my foundation, eyeshadow and lip brush, and anything that is used with a liquid or cream texture (it's not so important for brushes that are used with powders). I swoosh the bristles on some wet soap, rinse until they come clean and leave to dry flat Take care of your brushes, they're an investment.

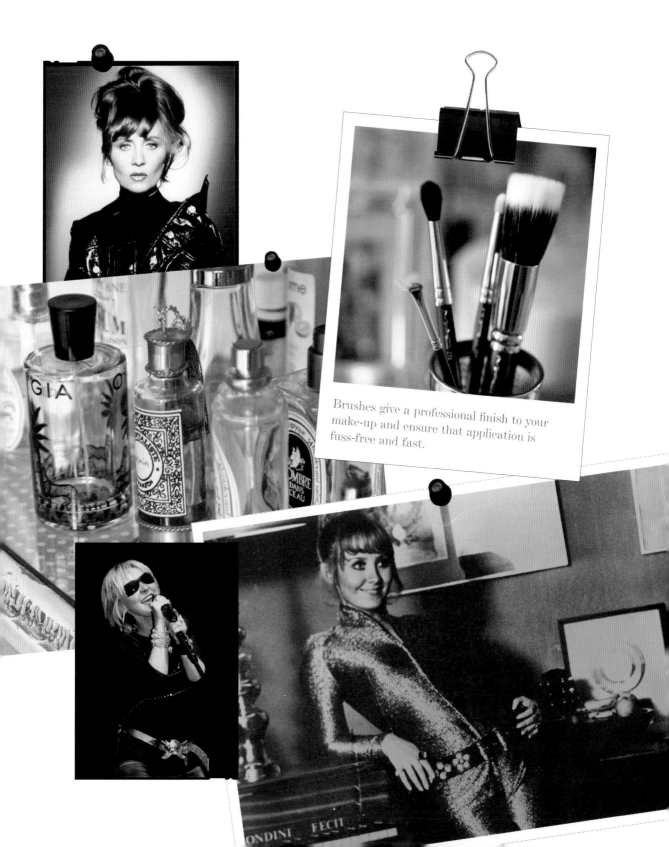

Brushes give a professional finish to your make-up and ensure that application is fuss-free and fast.

My *Go-anywhere* Kit

This is what's in my little Anya Hindmarch pouch that I keep in my handbag for daytime touch-ups. I've pared it right down because I just don't want to lug a great kit everywhere with me.

* My gorgeous jewelled butterfly magnifying mirror by Jay Strongwater— a gift from my very good friends Elton John and David Furnish. To be honest, when they first gave it to me, I wasn't sure I'd ever use it, but now I can't go anywhere without it. One side is magnifying, the other is 'normal' — and it gives a much better view of my make-up than the mirror in any palette. It's girly and feminine and I LOVE it!

* Two MAC lip pencils, my eye balm and my Dior Skinflash concealer. (Don't forget to wash the brush of this regularly.)

* A Lancôme Le Crayon Kôhl, snapped in half so that it fits in my kit.

* Shu Uemura twist-up powder brush. A brilliant, compact brush with its own lid to keep powder from going all over your kit. I don't want to carry powder around with me because it tends to spill all over everything. Disaster! But if I touch this into just a smidgen of powder that's in the lid of my compact, before I put the brush in my bag, there's enough still in the bristles to banish the shine from my nose when I touch up my make-up during the day.

* My fan-shaped blusher brush. I don't carry the blusher itself around with me; again, this brush has enough colour impregnated in the bristles to add just a little extra flush to my cheeks during the day. It's not like I'm going on safari!

What do people compliment you on?
Rosebud lips?
The colour of your eyes?
A beautiful smile?

Take your clue from that:
whatever friends mention is
probably your best feature,
so learn to play that up.

But don't obsess about 'flaws'.
Nobody else notices them: they
see the whole beautiful picture…

And, anyway, that's why
make-up was invented…

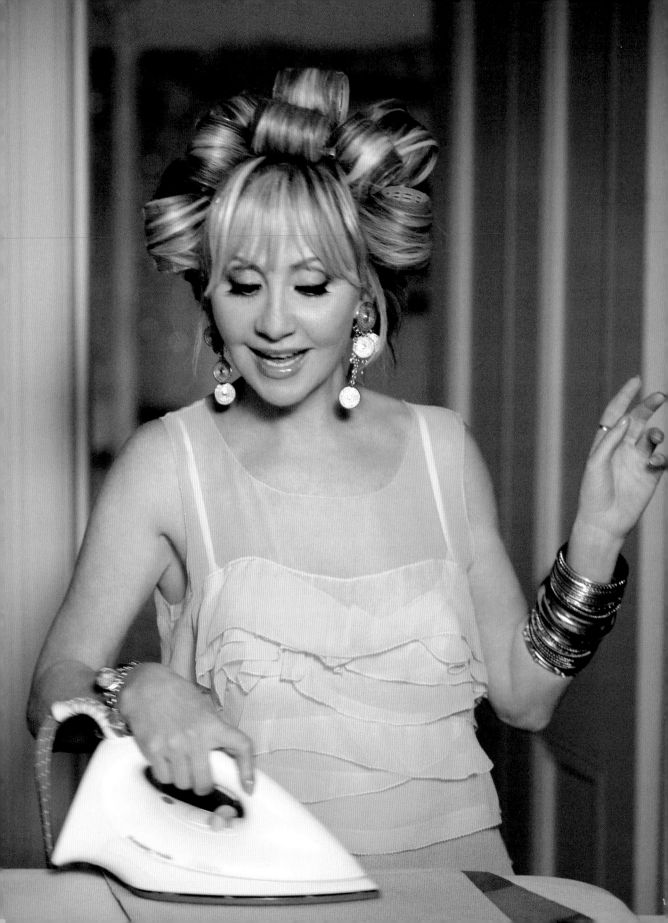

It's All About the Hair

A Good Hair Day
is a
Great Day

You know what? If I hadn't been a singer, I was desperate to be a hairdresser. I always used to give haircuts to the boys in my bands. I even cut Maurice Gibb's hair, when I was married to him, and I didn't do such a bad job, if you don't mind me saying so. Then later I even married a hairdresser — John Frieda, for heaven's sake! Well, everyone in my family said it was only appropriate that I finally had my own live-in hairstylist. They call me 'Hair Woman'. Everyone who knows me knows that I'm obsessed. And because of that, over the years I have had every hairstyle known to man — or rather, known to woman — and made every hair mistake, with (trust me) more than my share of bad hair days. I once went mad with a perm and had my very own Harpo Marx season (and those pictures are not my favourites!), and another disaster was my Mia Farrow pixie cut, by Leonard. Nightmare! I need a bit of oomph at the roots; that short haircut, cropped to the bone, just didn't work with my shape of face. But I only discovered that *afterwards*, unfortunately...

I've seen women burst into tears in the hairdresser's — and I've been that woman, on occasion, and felt like that (although I usually wait until I get home!) — because hair is so inextricably linked with how we feel about ourselves. A good hair day is a great day. A bad hair day? Pass the paper bag, honey! But hopefully, what I'm going to share with you here will mean that you can save your paper bags for your shopping, in future.

Time to get hair happy...

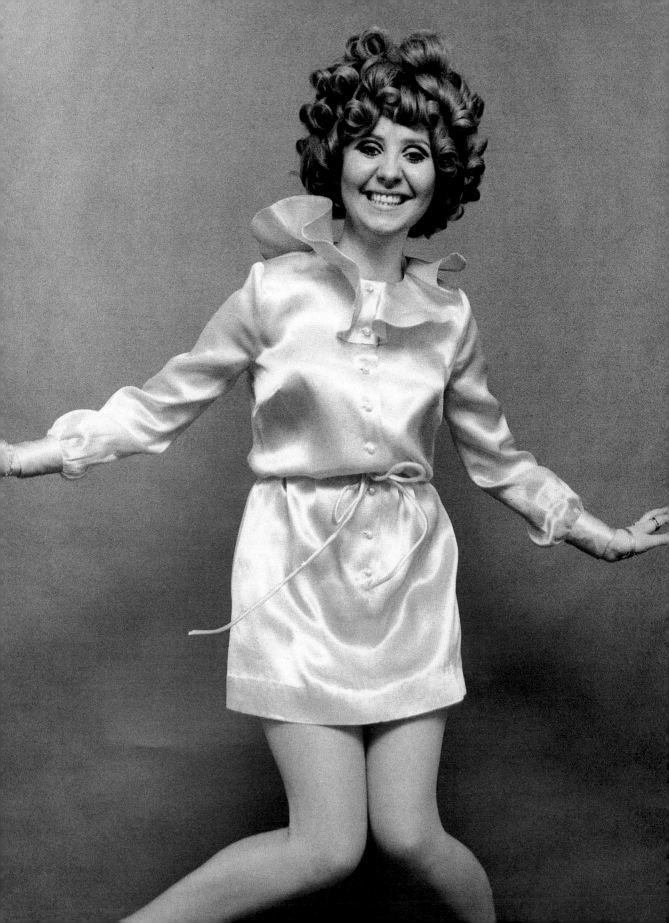

My Hair History

Now, I'm from the west side of Glasgow and I think maybe it's a Glaswegian thing to be so hair-obsessed: the cut, getting the style just right, it's like it's in our water, or the bread we eat. Where I come from in Glasgow, we were *so* fashion-conscious: working hard all week to buy something great to wear, getting our hair done at the weekends to go dancing... Back when I was growing up, hair was all about perms and rollers and sitting down in the hairdresser once a week — which I used to do with my lovely mum. My mum was obsessed with her hair. (She had even thicker hair than me. Actually, mine's quite fine but I'm lucky because there's lots of it.)

When she had it done, I'd critique her hair and tell her, 'I don't think that colour's quite right on you', because I was always looking and watching and figuring out what worked and what didn't.

When I came to London, Marion, my manager, took me in hand, image-wise. I thought she was terribly chic and sophisticated: She was your cashmere, high-heeled, Chanel sort of woman. An Astrakhan coat with a chinchilla collar, and shiny dark hair like Maria Callas. I aspired to that sort of chic, even though I was just 14 years-old! (Why is it we always want to look older when we're teenagers and when we're older we want to look younger?) There was a touch of the 'Eliza Dolittles' about it, with Marion as Henry Higgins. In hair terms that meant whisking me off to her friend Vidal Sassoon, at his original salon at Grosvenor House, to give me a new look.

This turned out to be my first — but not my last — paper bag moment at the hairdresser's. At the time Vidal was *the* hairdresser; he was doing Twiggy, and Mary Quant, and anyone in the 1960s who was anyone at all. His look was all about freeing women from backcombing and lacquer and beehives, and making hair swingy. Well, I was Little Miss Backcombing — because if I'd learned one thing, it's that I need a little height at the roots — but Vidal teased that out, plastered it down and flattened it to my head and went snip, snip, snip! He made it absolutely poker-straight, with a Jane Birkin fringe. When I looked in the mirror, all I could see were my chubby cheeks. I didn't think it was 'soft' or 'flattering' — and I wanted my backcombing back.

So Vidal created a lot of famous looks — but not for me. I went home and cried; I didn't have the greatest self-esteem, was always comparing myself (unfavourably) with the great beauties of the day — and really, that hairdo didn't help. What I realised is that it didn't *work* for me to be liberated from bigger hair. It doesn't suit me to have it plastered flat to my head, because I need a bit of root-lift; I need a bit of height. So I learned from *that* hair mistake.

It's all about striking a balance. If you have too much volume you can look mumsy or matronly. At the time, when I had tons of volume, I thought I looked *fa-bu-lous* — and it took me years of looking at pictures of myself to really understand what worked and what didn't. It was all part of my learning curve. (If you're not sure, ask your best and most trusted girlfriend what *she* thinks.) After Vidal, I used to go to Ricci Burns, who was famous for 'dressing' the hair — none of that wash-and-go stuff for Ricci.

'I THINK MAYBE IT'S A GLASWEGIAN THING TO BE SO HAIR-OBSESSED.'

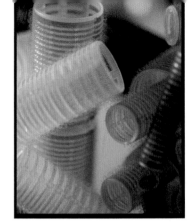

And he put me back in my comfort zone. Today, I understand that it's so crucial for women to have a great relationship with their hairdresser: someone you can trust, but someone who can also look at you with a fresh eye, every now and then, and suggest changes that update your look — but won't rock your world. Maybe you are lucky enough to have someone like that in your life right now. If not, then you need to find the best hairdresser you can.

Honestly, I believe that, in terms of spending priorities, it's more important to invest in your hair even than what you put on your body. Let's face it, most of your clothes languish in the wardrobe for most of the time — but your hair you wear every day, day in, night out! So if you haven't found your perfect hairdresser match, there are several ways to find him or her.

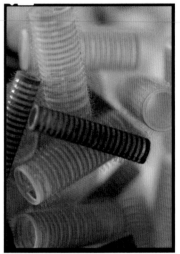

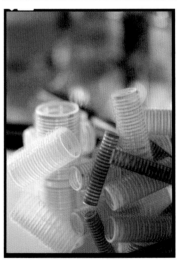

'BECAUSE IF YOU'VE GOT A BUSY LIFESTYLE, THERE'S ABSOLUTELY NO POINT HAVING A STYLE THAT'S GOING TO TAKE A LOT OF TIME TO RECREATE.'

Hair Envy

I wish I had the kind of hair — like my niece Tiffany — where I could get out of the shower, shake my head and look fabulous. (Hers is long and chestnut brown and *gorgeous*. I have serious hair envy with my niece Azalea, too!) Uh-uh. If I don't blow-dry mine, it gets half dry and turns to frizz.

First of all, ask a friend whose hair you like which hairdresser she goes to. If you see someone on the street whose hair you just love, don't feel shy to ask where they go to — I promise they'll be flattered rather than annoyed! (We *all* love to be complimented on our hair...) Then you can make an appointment to go along for a chat because, though they don't always shout it from the rooftops, all hairdressers offer free, brief consultations when you can talk through what you want, and your hair type, and how much time you have for maintenance. Because if you've got a busy lifestyle, there's absolutely no point having a style that's going to take a lot of time to recreate.

It is human nature to want what you don't have, in hair terms. So, you can either decide that you want to make a life's work out of your hair, to make it do what it doesn't want to do — straighten it if you're naturally curly, put curls in if it's poker-straight — or you can go with what nature gave you. If you're going to fight nature, then be prepared to put in the time (and investment in lots of product) to tame it. Personally, I decided a long time ago that it was better to 'go with the flow'. I've had perms — but as I've got older, my hair — happily — has developed a tiny bit more natural wave of its own, so I mostly go with that. (To help it out, I sometimes use tongs or heated rollers — not that great for the condition of the hair, but it's not something I do every day.)

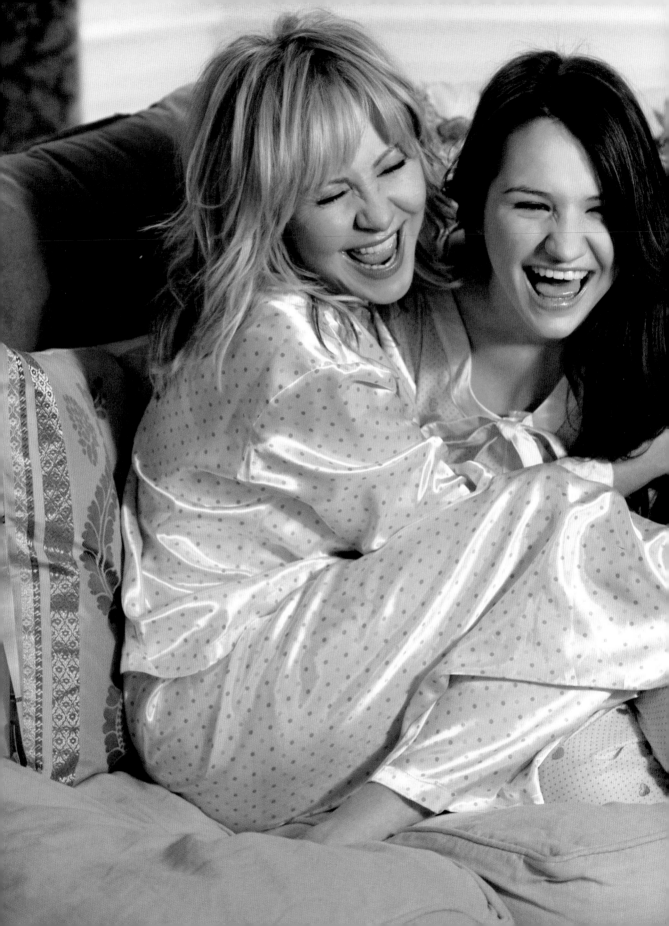

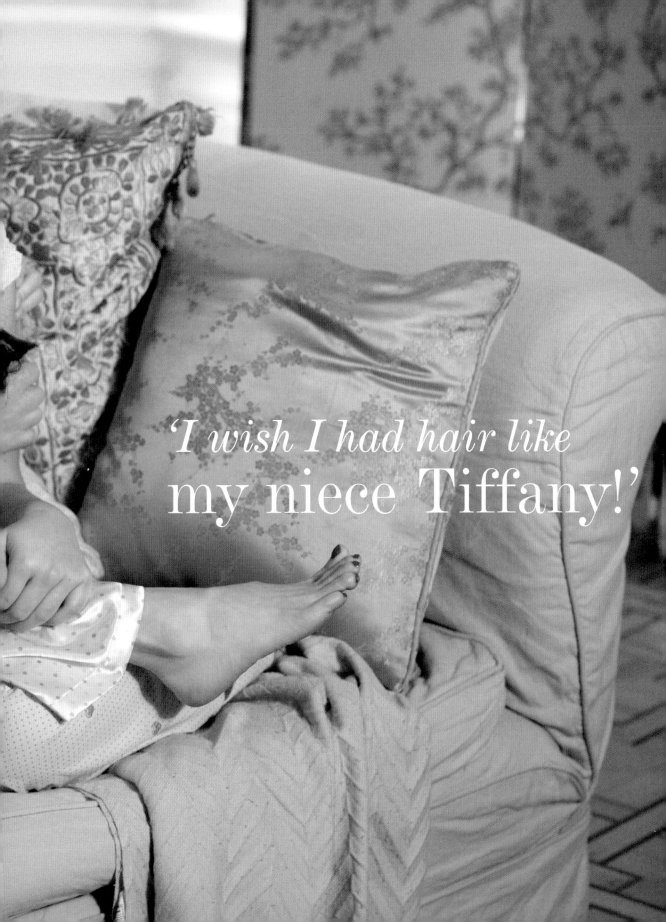

'*I wish I had hair like* my niece Tiffany!'

Lots of Layers

Layers are sexy and they give movement. I rather love that 'bed hair' look, as long as it isn't taken to extremes. If your style is all one length, having a few layers cut into it is a great way to experiment with something different without sacrificing the length completely. I absolutely do *NOT* subscribe to the idea that when you hit 40, long hair has to go — it all depends on the woman. My friend Peggy Lipton, the actress (who was married to Quincy Jones), has wonderful, straight long hair that looks fabulous. Jane Seymour still looks great with long, straight hair. It's harder if you've got bushy, wild hair — unless you're Diana Ross — or you can have your hair blow-dried all the time. Anyway, if you're going to keep your hair longer, it needs to be in great condition.

For many women, layers are the way to go to give it swing and shape. Even shorter hair needs some sway, some swing — otherwise hair can look a bit like a helmet. (But one other thing I do know is that nobody over 30 should have short layers cut in the top. It's one of the most ageing looks you can have. Even the Princess of Wales used to look a bit middle-aged when her top layers were too short. Layers are sexy, but they shouldn't be *too* short...)

'IF YOU'RE GOING TO KEEP YOUR HAIR LONGER, IT NEEDS TO BE IN GREAT CONDITION.'

Blow-drying

How often do I blow-dry my hair, or have it done? As little as possible — probably once a week. I do think that it's possible to be a little too fanatical about daily washing of hair (and all that extra time you have to spend styling it). American women, especially, are obsessed with having to shampoo and condition every single day. When I was younger, we certainly never washed our hair every single day — my mum made that blow-dry last a week, and I certainly don't wash my hair every day! (Honestly, I think there are more important things to spend my time on than doing my hair). I would encourage you to try — just to experiment — and see if you can leave your hair for a bit longer than usual —a few days, maybe —before washing it again. Try it. That's time we can all spend doing something we really enjoy, rather than beating our hair into submission (which is certainly the way it always feels for me. Mine has a tendency towards frizziness). Instead of doing your hair, you could be walking, working out or hanging out with your friends or family. If you save yourself half an hour a day, that's over a week a year!

And, in reality, most women, by the time we hit our forties, have left any scalp oiliness behind — it's part of the transformation of skin, and it's why so many of us suffer drier skin as the years roll by. So the scalp's usually 'normal', or a wee bit dry, and certainly doesn't need washing every day. In fact, the natural oils in hair are good for it — that's why they're there, for heaven's sake! They add a little body, and they are good for condition. I think it's really good to learn a few tricks that extend the time between hairdos. In between washes, I just play around with my hair: I'll pile it on my head, pull it back with a hairband, maybe tong it to put some curls back in.

Be Your Own Stylist

With haircuts, I really do believe that change is as good as a rest, too. If you're wondering how your hair would look with a different style, play with your hair in front of a mirror. Pile it up. Clip it. Pull it back. Ideally, have two mirrors: a big, well-lit mirror on the wall and a hand mirror, so that you can see yourself from different angles. Have a session where you really assess yourself, and what looks good. If you don't have the confidence to judge this for yourself, ask a friend whose opinion you trust. Or book a consultation with a hairdresser and get him or her to 'play' with your hair in front of the mirror. By holding your hair in different styles, they can pretty much 'fake' what a new look is going to be like on you, and that can take the fear factor out of having a new style. I sometimes find that a new stylist is a tiny bit afraid to try a different style on me — since a lot of people know that I was married to a hairdresser — but I tell them to go for it. If it doesn't work, I'll change it or chop it. I'm not afraid.

I really like change; I think it's so important not to get into a hair rut. At one point I even had a green flash in my hair, which looked a bit like a feather, just for fun. It's fabulous if you find a hairdresser that 'gets' you and you really have a rapport with — every woman needs one of those (though she doesn't necessarily have to marry him!). Teamwork is a wonderful thing when it comes to hair. But the challenge with some hairdressers is that, after a while, they start to see you in the same way. A good hairdresser nudges you towards a change of style occasionally, if he or she feels you need a fresh 'look'. If you feel you've been stuck with the same 'do' for too long, nudge your hairstylist instead.

Finding Rapport

It can sometimes help to take a photograph in, to show the stylist what you want. Most don't mind at all — it can be helpful to make sure you're speaking the same language (else there's a risk that if you say 'shorter', they might interpret that as a 'pixie cut', when you meant shoulder-length!). Sometimes you just need to switch to another stylist in the same salon. If your stylist goes on holiday, use the opportunity to try out someone else. (Trust me: they're quite grown-up about this; in salons, it comes with the territory.)

At my ex-husband John Frieda's salon, the stylists are sometimes encouraged to go to drawing classes or to study sculpture because it's so good for teaching them about bone structure, and to really assess what styles work for different face shapes. There's quite a science as to what will or won't suit you. For your guidance, I've picked the brain of Kevin Moss, my hairstylist at John Frieda, about the best cut for different faces — just turn the page and the wisdom's all there.

I haven't got a crystal ball so I can't tell what *your* face looks like — but Kevin's tips should give you some guidance, and maybe inspiration for a new look. Because the great thing about hair is that it does grow! Even a disastrous haircut grows out (though I hope you won't ever have one of those again). I think what I instinctively knew at a really young age — when I so longed to be a hairdresser — is that you can be really creative through hair. I've certainly been pretty creative with mine down the decades!

I've definitely had that burst-into-tears moment at the hair-dresser, but over the years I've learned what does and doesn't make me look great. And I plan to go on varying my look for the rest of my life. Shorter. Longer. Wavier. Straighter. Fringe. No fringe. Perhaps not a green flash again — but watch this space!

Your *Perfect* Haircut – It's All in the Face Shape

Having been married to a hairdresser for so many years — as well as being obsessed with hair from such an early age — I've spent quite a lot of time assessing why certain hairstyles look better on me, my girl pals and the women I see around me. You want to know what the secret is? It's getting a style that works with your own face shape and bone structure. If you don't do that, any style you have is going to look like it's been plonked on your head.

My hairstylist, Kevin, spends absolutely ages cutting my hair. *Ages!* Sometimes I want to get up out of the chair and run! But he has an amazing eye for bone structure and what works best. I asked Kevin to help me a little here —he's really the expert (and all credit where credit's due). Here are some great guidelines for what will be the most flattering haircut for you (and it might help explain some of those paper bag moments you've had in the past!).

The other essential factor you should take into consideration is your lifestyle, and the amount of time you've got for styling. As I've said, fighting nature takes time. Let your stylist know how much time and effort you're prepared to devote to upkeep. There's no point in him or her giving you a style that is going to be higher maintenance than you can manage, so be sure to communicate how often you wash your hair and how much time you can give it.

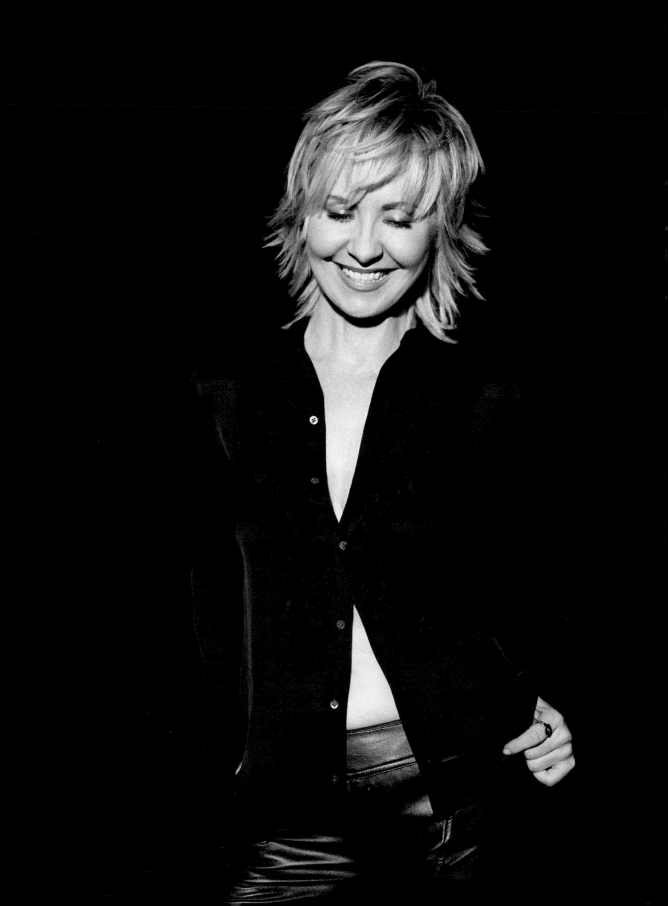

Do you have an *oval* face?

Lucky you! This is the one face shape that looks good with almost any haircut. Interestingly, pretty much *all* haircuts are designed to help achieve an oval face shape — to balance the face and give it the right proportions so it's not too long, or too square, but appears oval (which is considered the 'perfect' face shape — although, as you can tell by now, I'm not about perfection, but about bringing out the best in what *you've* got...). With this shape, you could even go very short — think Kylie, with her pixie cut — provided your jawline's still quite sharp.

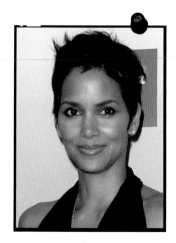

Do you have a *long* face?

Whatever you do, avoid a straight bob — but instead go for hair that flicks and kicks out at the jawline, away from the face. (If you also have a more pointed chin, you definitely want to avoid hair that curls under towards the chin, because it will just accentuate that.) Don't try to build too much height and volume at the crown, because that will also create the illusion that your face is longer and straighter than it is. Instead, why not experiment with a fringe? This can 'shorten' the face (but make sure the fringe is soft, rather than a solid line).

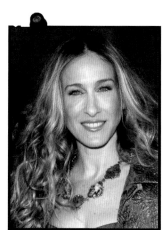

Do you have a *square* face?

Think of Angelina Jolie and Audrey Hepburn, who both fall into this category: they look best with their hair away from their face, showing off that amazing jaw-line. Sometimes a geometric cut looks great with this face shape. You can also experiment

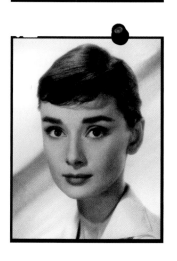

with different styles of fringe. a see-through fringe, or sometimes a fringe that's a bit graduated at the side — but never a fringe that's blunt and straight across, that's for sure. Otherwise, think gentle waves...

Do you have a *round* face?

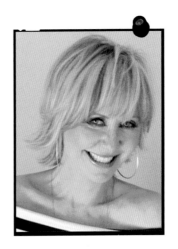

This is my face shape (although, just to complicate things, I also have a square jaw and a short head, which is an asset for photographs, and *great* with hats)! Anything too sleek to the head will give a pudding-basin effect, so you should be looking at something soft, choppy and textured. Layers work well with a round face — and if you can get them cut to your cheekbone-level, you can blow-dry them outwards at that point, which sort of creates the illusion of a more sculpted face. Add height and volume at the roots when you're blow-drying. And if you want a fringe (it works well with this face shape), have it graduated and cut a wee bit on an angle. If you feel that your neck is a bit on the plump side, or not as swan-like as you'd like it in your dreams, have your hairdresser break up the ends to create texture and softness. Avoid curls (as per my Harpo Marx phase!)

Do you have a *heart-shaped* face?

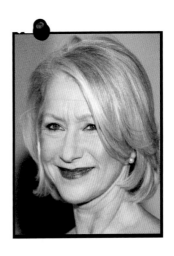

A heart-shaped face has a broad forehead and is narrower at the jaw. What your style should be trying to achieve is balancing the narrower jaw, with hair that kicks out, in choppy layers, to create volume lower down the face. A soft, graduated fringe is fantastic for this shape of face, because it softens the wider forehead.

The *Art* of Hair Styling

I often hear friends lament that their hair never looks as good when they do it themselves, at home, as when their stylist does it. Of course it would always help if we had an extra arm — in addition to the usual two — to achieve the perfect blow-dry but, trust me, even with two arms, it is possible if you know how... Again, Kevin gave me a little help with putting this into words, because he's such a pro — and I believe we should all tune into the wisdom of professionals, whenever we get the opportunity.

Get the moisture out

I like to apply product when it's completely wet, but don't attempt to style hair till it's at least 80 per cent dry, or you're just wasting your time and energy — and giving yourself arm-ache. (Either that, or you can end up with hair that's been 'over-styled', so all the oomph has gone out of it.) Ideally, squeeze and then blot hair dry with a towel and then use a hairdryer to ruffle it until it's basically just damp. If you want to achieve extra volume, hang your head upside-down — provided this won't make you dizzy; you may find it more comfortable to simply tilt your hair and blow the drier into it, which will also achieve that all-important 'lift' at the roots. (If you do let your hair get a touch too dry, then spritz it with a plant mister to put some moisture back in before styling.)

Apply your styling product

This is where you need a little help from your hairstylist, because he or she can tell you exactly what you need to use.

(Don't feel like they're just trying to sell you product; what they really want is for their handiwork to be shown off to its best advantage, and the correct product prescription helps with that.)

Massage the product through from roots to ends

Ideally, you want to section hair off and work the product through each section, rather than smoosh a whole load of product into one spot. (It can help to use clips to section hair, not just when applying product, but actually when drying the hair — which I'll get onto in a second.) Don't overload your hair with products: today's products are designed for maximum effect, without having to use masses of them — and when products don't work, it's often 'pilot error'! Read instructions and ask your stylist to show you how much of each product you should be applying. But failing that, a palmful of mousse, for instance, is about right for hair that is just above the shoulder, whereas a five-pence-sized dollop of gel — no more — is also enough for medium-length hair. A good way to apply it at home yourself is with a vent brush or a Denman brush: work the mousse through the brush, then brush through your hair. Don't apply directly to the hair itself or you'll end up with too much product in one place.

Use a good hairdryer

Invest in a powerful hairdryer with a directional nozzle. I know, I know: the nozzle's the bit everyone throws away when they buy a new hairdryer, but it's the most important bit! The more powerful the hairdryer, the quicker you'll get results. (Hairdressers can often be sweet-talked into ordering a professional hairdryer for you, which will help you achieve more professional results.)

Then start styling...

Again, my advice is to ask your stylist which brushes are right for you — they make all the difference in the world.

Do the front first

This frames your face, and it's the first (and often the only) bit that someone notices about your hairdo. Sometimes all it takes to refresh a style is to dampen down the area around the face and style it again. (It sure beats washing your hair and starting from scratch.) If you're doing your whole style, move from the front to the sides, top and then the back and underneath last.

Go with the flow...

For super-shiny results, blow-dry down the hair, from root to tip. This smoothes the cuticle and enhances the natural shine.

Give it a shot of cold air

This helps to 'set' the style, so it holds its shape much longer. (Think of how pliable plastic is when it's warm. Hair works the same; a sudden blast of cold air 'fixes' what you've done.)

Just add wax...

I love the textured finish that hair wax gives: choppy, modern and a million miles away from those stiff perms our mums wore. (And me, in my time!) You only need a smidgen, though. Put a dab in your hand, rub your palms together really well and run your fingers through your hair to create texture. Lift the hair at the roots, for volume, and twist the ends, for definition.

Or just add serum...

If you have the frizzies, serum works miracles. You need just the teensiest amount — the size of a five-pence coin — then rub your palms together and smooth over the hair. Some women can't live without serum, but even those who don't generally have frizzy hair can find it really useful on a tropical holiday, or when the weather's humid. The danger is that you end up with a lump, so start with a little, and repeat the process if necessary, rather than using a big dollop all at once.

When my hair isn't behaving itself I sling on my favourite hat and *voila*! Instant style points and not a hair out of place.

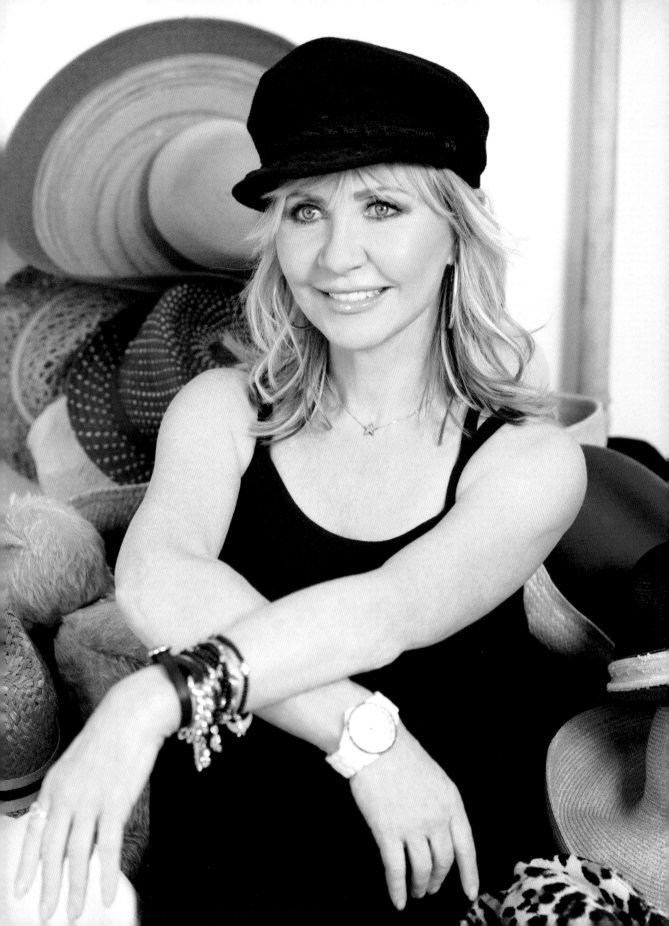

The Perfect Blow Dry

(with a little help from my hairdresser...)

If you have wash-and-go hair, thank your lucky stars. Because, for most of us, hair is higher maintenance than that. I am lucky: I'm able to go to the hair salon to have blow-dries, but my hairdresser Kevin Moss has drilled into me the secret of blow-drying my own hair. This is what I've learned, but it might be different for you.

Show and Tell

My best — my very *best* — piece of advice is to ask your stylist how to do your hair at home. Get him or her to show you the tricks, the products, the brushes and even the hairdryer that will give the best results. It's like making the most of the investment you've made in a good cut. Trust me: you'll get far more out of your hour in the hairdresser if you pick your stylist's brains about hairdrying technique than if you sit with your nose in a copy of *OK!*

Move That Scalp

I think you have to keep everything movin': your body, your mind, your face, your spirit — and your scalp! That's what my friend Joyce does: she really massages her scalp. It gets the blood flowing (and the brain, I'm convinced), and it lets all those nutrients get to the roots, which is terrific for hair health. I've taken to copying her.

The skin on the scalp is really an extension of the skin on the face, so it deserves its own generous helping of TLC. Did you know that you carry a lot of tension in your scalp? If you're really anxious about something, then it can be almost impossible to move the skin of the scalp over the skull. Try it! If your scalp is loose and moveable, then it's a sign that you're pretty chilled. That's the ideal. Massage it daily, not just when you're shampooing. Your hair — and your scalp — will love you for it.

Short to *Long*

I *l-o-v-e* hair extensions. I have the lowest boredom threshold with hair of just about anyone you can imagine. The wonderful thing about extensions, though, is that when you just absolutely HAVE to have longer hair, and you want it NOW — well, you can. If you look at just about anyone in Hollywood or any model in *Vogue*, they've got hair extensions. But you'd never know it, because the technology is so good these days that it just looks like great, lustrous, natural hair.

Now, once upon a time, the bonds at the roots that attached the extensions were clunky and uncomfortable, but the technology has improved tremendously. Nowadays, extensions are what my niece Azalea calls 'boyfriend-friendly': in other words, the man in your life can run his fingers through your hair and he won't even notice the extensions are there.

When I was first in London, it was all about hairpieces. Hairdressers like Alexandre de Paris and Ricci Burns used to create these amazing, elaborate looks, piling up fake hair on the head. To my mind, hair extensions are the contemporary equivalent of those hairpieces. It doesn't have to be a huge investment.

Thinning Hair

Extensions are really a godsend for women with naturally thin or thinning hair — which can be stress-related or hormone-related — because they add volume and oomph. And that can really boost a woman's confidence, because I know that thinning hair knocks your self-esteem for six. Now, they aren't cheap, but if you're feeling like you can't face the world because your hair's too thin — and I do understand that there are plenty of women who feel like that — then extensions absolutely have to be worth the investment. (In fact, as a cheaper alternative, you can now get inexpensive clip-in ones, and apply them yourself.)

I have them done from time to time depending on my 'look' and because I'm a wee bit greedy and I just want more of it! I go to Connect, in Chalk Farm in London. (Victoria Beckham, Cheryl Cole and the Duchess of York have all had their extensions done there — as well as a long list of actors in those epics where the men have to have long hair.)

I warn you, though: hair extensions can be addictive...

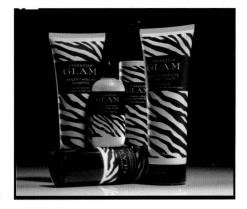

My Operation Glam hair products have all the vital ingredients for feel-good hair.

What You'll Find in My *D-I-Y Hair Kit*

OK, you may sense a little bias here. But these are truly the products that I use because I do think that John Frieda — who I originally met in the chair when he did my hair — makes absolutely incredible products at very, very accessible prices. So, here are the products and the tools that help make every day a good hair day...

* Operation Glam Larger-Than-Life Shampoo and Conditioner for fine to normal hair. If you weren't blessed with naturally glamorous hair, you need products that can help you look like you were! I need a little help to make my fine hair look full, so I use a shampoo that makes my hair look thicker and a conditioner that won't weigh my hair down. I also use a thickening product called Glammunition which really transforms my hair. The key is finding the right products for your hair type.

* A Mason-Pearson brush. This is the type your granny used to recommend, for those ritual 100 strokes a night. Well, I certainly don't do that, but I do *love* the feeling of the brush stimulating my scalp. It's a bit like massaging the scalp with the fingers: I feel like all those nutrients are flooding to the roots to make my hair healthy.

✳ Velcro rollers — a genius invention because (unlike in the 'old days') you don't need pins with these; just wind the hair round them to add extra volume. (You can blast with a hairdryer if you like, for more staying power.)

✳ Round styling brushes in different sizes, including a small one to lift the roots and add movement.

✳ Hair ties and hair 'claws'. You know what? A lot of the time I just want my hair up and out of the way, away from my face. So I pull it back and secure it with one of these. The secret at our age is not to pull too tight, but to make the hair look a bit soft and with a bit of height — that's what makes the difference between harsh and flattering.

✳ Kirby grips (remember them?). You can use them to pin your hair up, or — if you've added a little body with rollers or tongs — you can pin that oomph in place with invisible grips.

✳ I have a *great* collection of hats — loads of them — for when my hair's beyond redemption. My favourite is a peaked cap which I found in a shop near Topshop at Oxford Circus (see the picture on p.93!), and I just can't tell you how often people ask me where I got it. Check out shops like Accessorize — they have *excellent* soft hats — and spend some time in front of the mirror, just trying them on, playing with them, pulling bits of hair out and generally experimenting until you find a bad hair day hat (or three). It's what teenagers do. Why not? (It used to be all about baseball caps, of course, but I'm rather over them. Those really do look like you're trying to cover up bad hair...)

Blonde Ambitions

I always, always wanted blonde hair. My brother Billy, who is 18 months younger than me — had amazing Shirley Temple curls, and people would stop my mother in the street and say how pretty he was. I was constantly comparing myself (unfavourably) with him, because that's just how I am. It's where my longing to be blonde started. People would stop my mum in the street and say, 'Isn't she GORGEOUS?' and I'd stamp my foot and have a tantrum and say, 'He's a BOY, he's not a *girrrrlll!*' My mum even used to say she married my dad because he had curly hair and she'd have curly-haired blonde children — but not me. Oh, no. It's become naturally wavy now, but when I was little, it was mousy and straight and I had serious hair envy of my brother.

I have come to terms with the fact that I am naturally mousy. Of course, everyone used to think I was a natural redhead because by the time I recorded my first single, I'd been red for years. I used to go to the salon with my mum every Saturday to hang around while she had her weekly shampoo and set, and I was just desperate to be grown-up, like her. So first of all, I had my ponytail chopped off. And then — because my natural colour was really mousy, and I just hated it — I asked for a rinse. *A rinse!* But it turned out bright auburn, and I became a redhead, just like that.

I guess my hair was lighter than I'd thought it was, and it just soaked up the colour. And when I went into school on the Monday morning, my headmistress had a go at me in front of the whole class, and said, 'Marie, if you think that's going to attract the boys, you're absolutely wrong.' Well, my face turned the same colour as my hair — but by then, I was stuck with it.

I could get away with vibrant red hair when I was young, but as I've got older I've had to soften the colour to suit my skin tone.

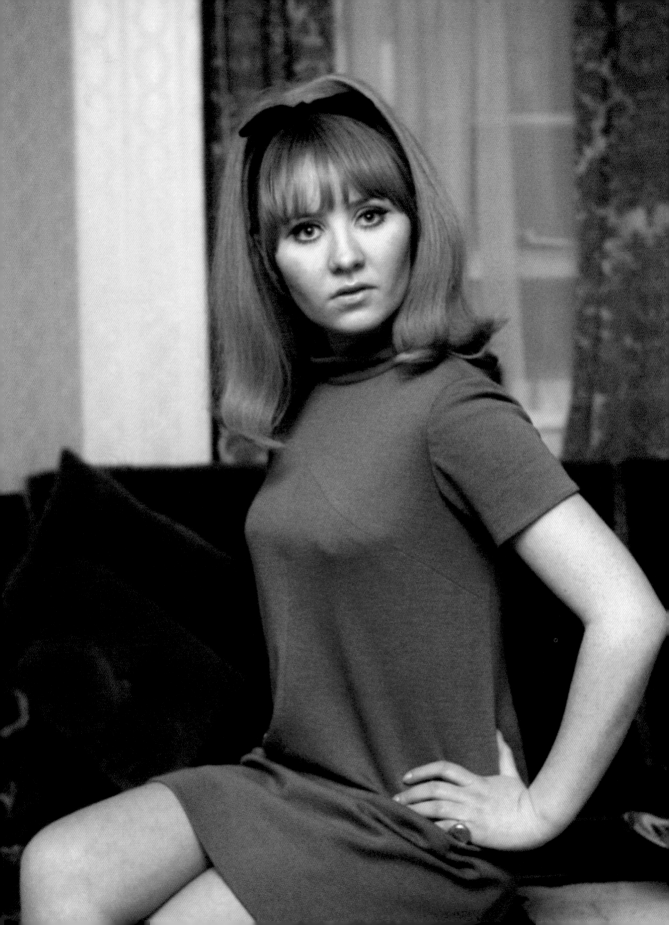

And the longer I had red hair, the more I began to like it. I had a really gorgeous aunt — one of my mother's sisters — who had red hair, and I thought it looked really attractive. So maybe there's a natural redhead in my DNA somewhere because, actually, it worked well with my skin tone. And, of course, it became my signature. I had green eyes and people thought I was fiery and passionate, so it suited my temperament.

When I arrived in London, I met some really great colourists, and over the years it's been every shade of red and quite a few shades of blonde. Quite a few years ago now — can it really have been 1985? — I was in the TV series of *The Secret Diary of Adrian Mole* (stepping into Julie Walters' shoes, which, let me tell you, was pretty scary), playing Adrian's mum, Pauline. I had to go dark, and after the series finished, I really felt like a change from being a redhead. It was the time when the supermodels were at their most super, and Linda Evangelista had this great look called 'The Skunk', with great stripes of white and black hair. So I copied her, and I realised that the lighter chunks really suited me. And eventually I became a blonde. And blonder. And *even* blonder. And I wish I'd known when I was 12 or 13 that, actually, it's absolutely the best colour for me.

Choose Colour Carefully

What I realised was that as I got older — and I think it's true for everyone — the red started to look harsh with my complexion. And if you've got even a slight tendency to redness, or rosacea, it's going to intensify that in your colouring. It got harder and harder to get the colour right, but blonde was much easier. It's a rule of thumb: as you age, your hair colour needs to go a few shades lighter than your natural tone to be flattering. Even if you once had jet-black hair, after a certain age you need to have some highlights to lift the colour — not blonde,

just a few shades lighter — or go lighter all over, like a warm
chestnut-brown. And with blonde, think cool shades like
cream and ivory — there shouldn't be any warmth or red in
there, because it'll look brassy. (And again, it'll pick out any
redness in your complexion, which is something we want to
avoid at all costs.)

Of course re-growth is an issue. If you have grey in your hair,
you'll probably want to opt for home hair-colouring because the
maintenance will be ouch-expensive in a salon. Hair-colouring
fixtures in the chemist's can be baffling, so if there's any way you
can twist your colourist's arm to recommend a product you can
use for keeping up your colour at home, then sweet-talk them
into doing that! Otherwise, always make a point of choosing a
semi-permanent version of a shade, or a rinse, the first time.
Don't go for a permanent colour, because that way tears lie...
Until you're *sure* it's the right shade for you. (Some of the big
hair-colouring brands, usefully, offer the same shade in semi-
permanent and permanent. You just want to triple-check at the
hair-colouring fixture that you've picked up the one you want.)

Blonde highlights are really tricky to do yourself, if you're
not a pro — but, actually, although you spend longer in the
chair having them done (so long, sometimes, that you want to
run screaming from the salon!), you make up for that with the
fact they're lower maintenance. A bit of dark re-growth with
highlights can even look sexy, I think. (Look at Madonna; she's
never been shy of her roots.) But if you've got highlighted or
blonde hair with grey re-growth, the good thing is that it's
barely noticeable for a while, because the tones are similar.
I certainly don't think any more that you need to panic if you
cut yourself some slack and leave it a week or two longer
than usual between hair-colouring sessions. I think that we can
all thank our lucky stars to be living in times when re-growth
looks hip — not like you've lost the plot and let yourself go!

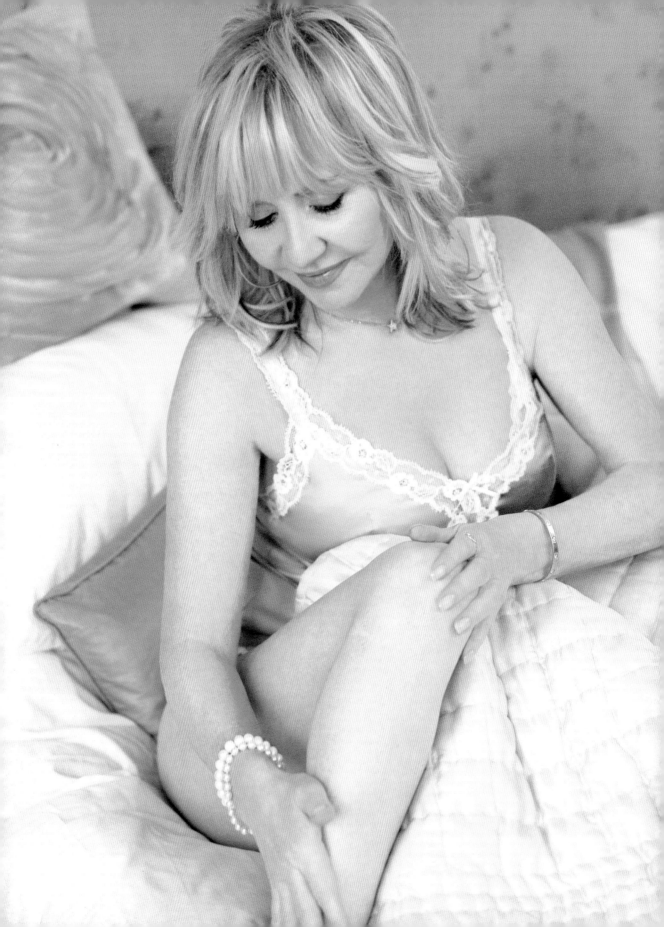

Bombshell Body

The Body
Beautiful

The absolute golden rule — at any age, but especially after 40 —
is to keep on movin'. Many of us have got into the habit of
working out, over the years, because we still wanted to be able
to zip up a favourite pair of jeans, or to make sure the waistband
of our favourite little black dress didn't get too tight. And, yes, of
course that's still important! But there is another really good
reason to work out: if we keep at it, exercise keeps us flexible
and strong. You know how little old ladies tend to fall straight
over, like ninepins? That's because when you're stiff, you often
become unsteady and fall over like a toy soldier — and that's
when bones and hips get broken. If you're flexible, you fall in a
completely different way. Depressing to think about? Well, a
wee bit, of course. But I certainly don't plan to be relying on a
Zimmer frame in my old age, honey. *Not* a good look on stage!

In the past I've done Jane Fonda's aerobics — and been burned out by the boredom. I've been a serious gym bunny and done circuit-training (and I still work out a couple of times a week, and do some weights for stamina, as you'll see in a minute). I've gone running — until my knees squealed in protest. Basically, now I mostly do a combination of yoga, some weights and walking — my dogs make sure I do plenty of that. (If you haven't got the motivation to get yourself out of the house, get a dog! Best trainer you can have!) And because I'm incapable of keeping my feet still for long, I dance, dance, dance!

To be honest, until I had my son Jordan, I didn't really work out at all: my work was so physical that I didn't really need to. Then gravity kicked in! My body isn't the way it used to be — that's just not achievable for anyone. But, with a little persistence and vigilance, you can still have a great body for your age. At *any* age...

'MY IMPERFECTIONS AND FAILURES ARE AS MUCH A BLESSING FROM GOD AS MY SUCCESSES AND MY TALENTS, AND I LAY THEM BOTH AT HIS FEET.'

Mahatma Gandhi

Say 'Yes' to Yoga

In the 1980s I found that the exercise that works absolutely best for me is yoga. John Lennon tried to get me into it almost 20 years before that — and meditation, which I'll get onto in a minute — but I guess I just wasn't ready. I remember Cleo Laine telling me in the late 1960s that she did yoga every single day of her life — and looked fabulous for it — but it still took me a while to catch on.

At first I used to pick up books on yoga in the quirky little health food shops I went into, when I was trying to track down the natural foods that made me feel so good. There would always be a bookshelf of self-improvement titles which I'd find myself flicking through, amid all the brown rice and miso soup. Since then, I've had some fabulous yoga teachers — especially my friend Bridget Woods Kramer, and Anna Ashby.

I don't do fashionable: no Bikram (think: hot, sweaty rooms), no *astanga* (which is a fast-paced type of yoga that everyone seems to be into. It was actually devised in India for young *brahmin* boys, who are ten years old, slim-hipped and have boundless

'THE JOURNEY OF A THOUSAND MILES BEGINS WITH A SINGLE STEP.'

Lao-tse

excess energy to burn off. That's why it doesn't work well for women's bodies, and I'm convinced that is why so many women I know end up getting injured by doing *astanga*). The type of yoga I'm into — and which seems to work for lots of women I know — is gentler, slower-paced and really restorative. I know that I can rely on a yoga session to get me back on my feet and get all the energy flowing when I'm exhausted.

I do my stretches a bit like a cat, anywhere and everywhere: backstage, on a plane, sitting on the sofa at home in front of the TV, circling my ankles, stretching out my calves. I get some *very* strange looks at 37,000 feet, but it does help with that in-flight puffiness, as well as stiffness from being cramped in an airline seat. If I'm going on stage, my stretches are as important as my vocal exercises, and I always do them before getting out of a car on a long journey, to loosen up my hips. I'll tell you a secret: I love my downward dog position so much that I could pretty much stay like that all day (and the increased blood flow from hanging your head upside-down is great for the skin and hair, too, because it boosts circulation). I asked my yoga teacher, Anna Ashby, for some easy stretches and positions that you can do at home (see pp.113–125) — but there are so many classes in every town now that it's easy to find one that works with your diary: early morning, lunchtime, after the family has gone to bed. No excuse not to!

I am really not surprised that yoga has now become one of the most popular forms of exercise all over the world, having spread far and wide from India, where it began around 7,000 years ago. It's amazingly strengthening, relaxing and flexibility-boosting — as well as tummy-flattening (always a good thing). But believe me: it is not just for skinny minnies. It's good whatever your shape and size. (And there are no rules that say you have to wear tight leotards or singlets: you'll be just fine in a pair of loose tracksuit bottoms and a baggy T-shirt — though you might want to tuck that in, once you progress to a shoulder-stand!)

HERE ARE MY GOLDEN RULES...

Little and often is better than a burst of occasional activity
That's how injuries happen. Even if you just do five minutes a day of yoga — stretching when you get up in the morning and last thing at night before bed, on a mat that you keep rolled up under your bed — that's better than nothing.

Don't let anyone push you further than you want to be pushed
Sometimes a teacher will try to stretch you, to help you get deeper into a posture (they often call them *asanas*, which is the Sanskrit word). Don't ever let them hurt you or feel too shy to say, 'No', or 'Stop!' There's no reason why yoga should hurt (other than a gentle, satisfying ache, occasionally, when you know you've had a good workout). You know your body better than anyone: trust it.

It's not a competition

Everyone's flexibility is different: we're stiff and/or bendy in different places, depending on whether we spend our lives sitting down, or standing in a shop, etc. Do only what your body allows you to do, which means trying not to pay attention to the girl at the front of the class who can not only touch her toes but almost gets her elbows on the ground. This is about you and you only!

Find a teacher you like

As I say, there are classes all over the place. But I've found that the important thing is to find someone who you feel is on your wavelength, and that you like — and that way, you'll want to go to class. But if that's just not practical, there are some really good DVDs that you can follow at home.

It's never too late to learn

And there is always something more to learn in yoga. I may have been doing this for 25 years and pretty much know my way around all 84 *asanas*, but I am still curious to discover more. And what I also like is that this is a form of exercise that you never, ever have to give up. Some of the greatest Yogis in the world still actively practise in their eighties and nineties and are as flexible as ever. What a great advertisement for such a wonderful form of exercise!

But do mix it up

Only yoga, or only walking, or only tennis or squash isn't enough for a fabulous shape, I'm afraid. Besides, you'll get bored. So on pp.128–147, let me show you how else I keep moving, active and healthy...

My Yoga

I regularly do yoga with the wonderful Anna Ashby – and the sequence always includes the poses that follow. These yoga poses can be done individually, or 'flowing' (one after the next) into one another. You will need a blanket, a strap and a rubber mat. Of course, if you have a medical condition or injury, it goes without saying: please consult your doctor before starting a yoga regime.

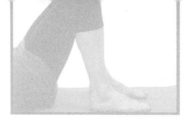

LIE FLAT WITH KNEES BENT
(five to ten minutes)

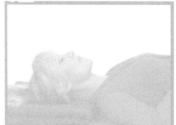

Benefits: Calming; deepens breathing; shifts focus inwards; releases tension in the back, shoulders, neck and belly; creates a sense of inner space

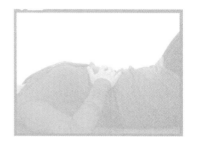

Props: Blanket and yoga mat

1   Lie on your back with your knees bent. Place a folded blanket underneath your neck and head.
2   Adjust your shoulder blades down your back, so that your shoulders soften and move back towards the floor and your chest broadens and lifts.
3   Push the flesh of your buttocks downwards towards your heels to lengthen the lower back.
4   Place your hands lightly on the front of your body, at your solar plexus (located just above your navel and below your sternum) and close your eyes.
5   Become aware of your breathing. Expand the breath into your hands, allowing your breath to become deeper and move through your entire body.
6   Allow yourself to relax deeper into the floor with each exhale. Relax the muscles of your face, your eyes and your tongue.
7   Keep your mind focused on the breath and let go of any thoughts of the past or future; rest in the present moment.

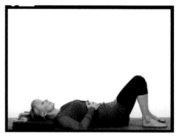

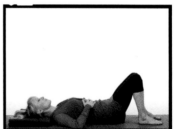

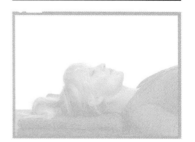

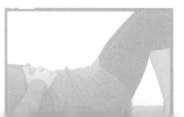

KNEES TO CHEST

Benefits: Massages the muscles of the back, releasing unnecessary tension

Props: Blanket and yoga mat

1   Lie on your back with your head supported on the blanket. Draw your knees into your chest. Clasp your hands below the knees.
2   First, allow your back to relax into the floor. Soften your shoulders back and widen the area across the top of your chest. Gently lengthen the back of your neck, keeping your chin level.
3   Now, begin to gently rock from side to side, breathing deeply (so that it feels as if the breath is moving into your back) as you rock for as long as you like.
4   Softly come back to centre and release, lowering your feet slowly to the floor.

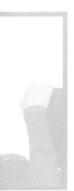
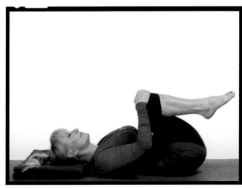
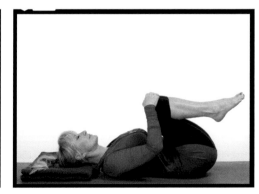

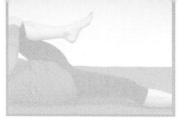

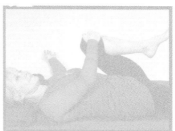

RECLINING TWIST

Benefits: **Releases tension in the back and spine; opens the shoulders; gently massages the internal organs in the body**

Props: **Blanket and yoga mat**

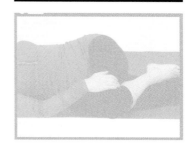

1 Lie on your back with your head supported on the blanket. Draw your left knee into your chest, and extend your right leg down onto the floor, with your toes pointing upwards. Clasp your hands just below your bent knee.

2 Imagine that you are pressing your right foot into a wall. Soften your shoulders back, lengthen your neck and breathe deeply, picturing the breath moving into your hip.

3 Open your left arm straight out to the side, palm facing upwards. Continue to hold onto your left knee with your right hand.

4 Inhale softly and, on the exhale, draw your left knee across your body and twist over to the right. Allow the back of the pelvis to come away from the floor as you twist over.

5 Draw your left shoulder back towards the floor. Don't force your shoulder or knee.

6 Look straight up towards the ceiling.

7 Lengthen your torso by lifting your chest and drawing your outer left hip downwards.

8 Breathe softly and evenly along the spine for a few breaths and, on an inhale, come up.

9 Repeat on the other side.

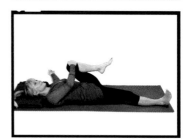

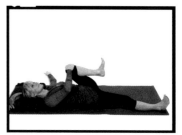

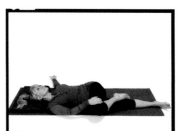

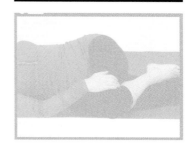

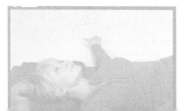

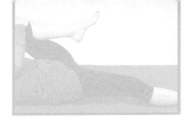

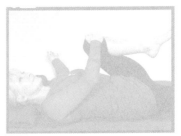

RECLINING FOOT-TOE POSE

Benefits: **Stretches the hamstring muscles at the back of the thigh; opens the hips; helps to release the diaphragm for a deeper breath**

Props: **Blanket, strap and yoga mat**

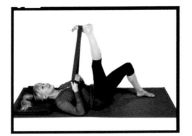

1   Lie on your back with your knees bent and your head supported on the blanket. Bend your right knee into your chest and place a strap just below the ball of the right foot.

2   Holding the strap lightly in both hands, stretch your right leg upwards until your leg is comfortably straight. (This may be lower than you think!)

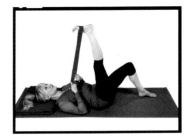

3   Soften your shoulders back towards the floor and lengthen your neck. Keep the back of the pelvis evenly resting on the floor.

4   Softly firm the top leg so that the muscles are engaged and then extend the foot upwards into the strap. Spread your toes and press your foot into the strap.

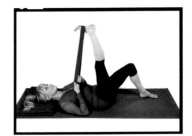

5   Breathe smoothly and evenly, relaxing the muscles of your face, eyes and tongue. Sustain the pose for at least five steady, even breaths.

6   Release your leg down and change sides. Repeat on the other side.

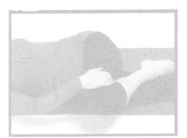

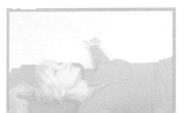

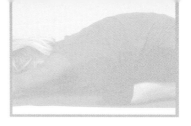

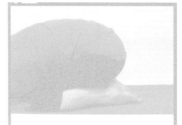

CHILD'S POSE

Benefits: **Calming; releases the hips; stretches the tops of the feet and the knees; stretches the spine; opens the shoulders**

Props: **Yoga mat and possibly a blanket**

1   Get onto all fours. Place your toes together and your knees apart (forming a 'V'). Sit back onto your heels (resting your buttocks against your heels) as you slowly 'walk' your hands forward and rest your forehead on the ground. (If your head doesn't touch, support it with the blanket. If your buttocks don't reach your heels or there is pain in your knees, place a blanket between your buttocks and heels for support. If the tops of your feet are tight, place a rolled-up blanket underneath them.)

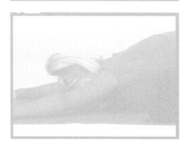

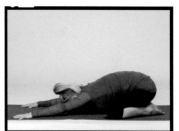

2   Draw back through your hips and stretch your arms forward. As you are stretching your arms, part your hands so that your little fingers are near the edge of your mat.

3   Spread your palms and firmly press your hands down, especially the inner edges of your hands.

4   Widen the area across your chest and soften and lengthen the back of your neck.

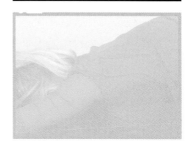

5   Breathe smoothly and evenly into your back. With each exhale, relax your forehead a little more against the floor and extend your arms a little further forwards.

6   On an inhale, slowly walk your hands back towards your body and sit back upright.

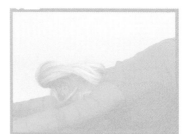

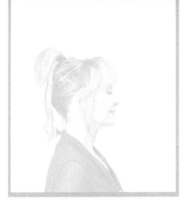

THUNDERBOLT POSE ARMS OVERHEAD

Benefits: **Stretches the tops of the feet, the shins and the knees; lengthens the torso; opens the shoulders and stretches the wrists and fingers**

Props: **Yoga mat and possibly a blanket**

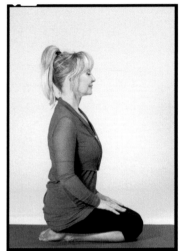

1   Get onto all fours with your feet and your knees hip-distance apart. Sit back onto your heels so that your buttocks are resting on your heels and your toes are pointing straight back (as described on p.117). Place your hands on your thighs. (If there is pain in your knees, place a blanket between your buttocks and heels for support. If the tops of your feet are tight, place a rolled-up blanket underneath them.)

2   Line up your shoulders over your hips and roll your shoulders back so that your chest is 'open' and relaxed. Softly lengthen the back of your neck so that your chin is level and relax your gaze.

3   Interlace your hands in front of you, rotate your wrists to extend your palms forwards and, on an inhale, stretch your arms up and over your head.

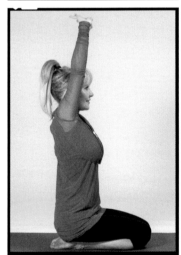

4   Gently lengthen your tailbone down to anchor your spine as you reach upwards, stretching through your wrists.

5   Again, soften and lengthen the back of your neck, relax your eyes and take smooth, even breaths.

6   After five breaths, release your arms down along your sides, maintaining the length of the torso. Change the interlace of your fingers (so if your right thumb was on top, you should now switch so that your left thumb is on top) and repeat.

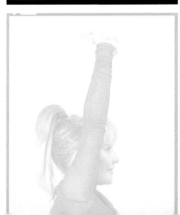

DOWNWARD-FACING DOG

Benefits: **Calming; general warm-up for the body; opens the shoulders; lengthens the hamstrings; strengthens the arms and legs; gentle inversion**

Props: **Yoga mat**

1   Get onto all fours with feet and knees at hip-distance apart.
2   Place your hands on the floor, one-hand's distance in front of your shoulders, but slightly wider than your shoulders, lining up your little fingers with the edge of your mat. Ensure that your index fingers are parallel. Check that your knees are just behind and in line with your hips.
3   Firm your arms by spreading out your palms and rooting your hands against the floor.
4   Curl your toes underneath you, spreading the weight across your toes.
5   Inhale. On the exhale, press yourself back so that your buttocks are almost resting on your heels, like the child's pose with your toes curled under. Walk your hands slightly forward so that your arms are straight and grounded.
6   Inhale. On the exhale, lift your knees up from the floor, keeping your arms strong.
7   With the knees still bent, press yourself back and up, lifting your buttocks. Soften the neck and release your head.
8   Slowly straighten your legs, pressing your thighs back and stretching your heels back. Stretch your arms forward, rooting your palms into the mat.
9   Take five smooth, even breaths as you sustain the pose and. release on an exhale coming down into Child's Pose. Rest.

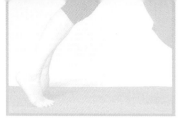
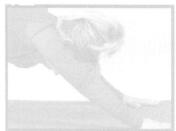
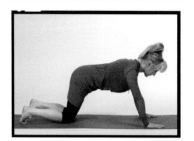
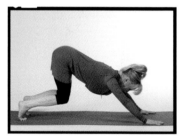
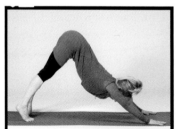
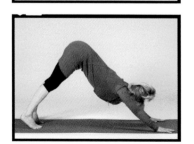
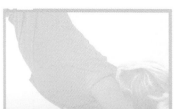

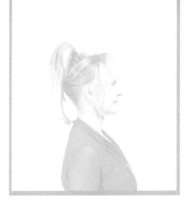

MOUNTAIN POSE

Benefits: **Grounding; centring; promotes optimal posture; strengthens the feet and the legs**

Props: **Yoga mat**

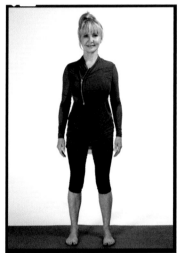

1. Place yourself in the centre of your mat, so that the mat is oriented width ways.
2. Place your feet hip-width apart and release your arms so they hang by your sides.
3. Line up the inner edges of your feet and spread out your toes evenly. Press down through the four corners of your feet.
4. Move your weight back a little so that you move towards the front of your heels, rather than on the balls of your feet.
5. Gently firm your legs as if you were squeezing a wood brick in between your inner thighs. It should feel as if your leg muscles are firming into the bone, creating a stabilising effect.
6. Press the tops of your thighs back and softly lengthen your tailbone down, balancing your pelvis.
7. Gently lengthen your spine upwards as you stretch back down through your feet.
8. Widen across the top of your chest and gently move your shoulders back. Softly lengthen the back of your neck.
9. Line up your ankles, hips, shoulders and ears in a vertical line as much as possible.
10. Keeping the legs firm, relax your fingers, your tongue and your solar plexus. Breathe fully and deeply.
11. Keep your eyes on the horizon line, but relax your gaze.
12. Standing tall, feel as if you are grounded to the floor and rooted like a mountain, ascending upwards towards the sky.

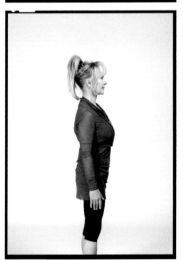

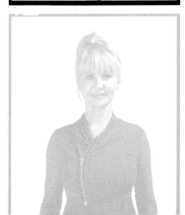

UPWARD-REACHING HAND POSE

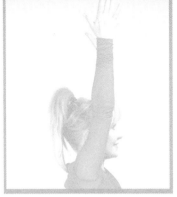

Benefits: Grounding; opens the shoulders; extends the trunk

Props: Yoga mat

1 Stand in the mountain pose in the centre of your mat, so that the mat is oriented width ways.
2 Align your mountain pose according to the instructions on the opposite page.
3 On an inhale, sweep your arms up and over your head. Keep your hands shoulder-width apart and roll your thumbs to point back.
4 As you root down through your feet, softly stretch up through and beyond your fingertips.
5 Relax your tongue and soften and lengthen your neck.
6 Imagine that your arms begin at the sides of your ribcage as you stretch upwards, lengthening the sides of the ribcage.
7 Take five smooth, steady breaths.
8 On an exhale, release your arms down by your sides.

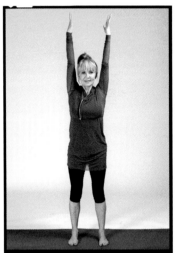

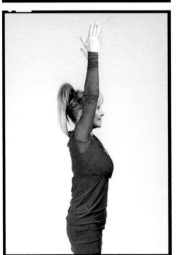

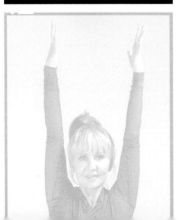

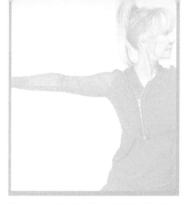

WARRIOR POSE II

Benefits: Grounding; invigorating; opens the hips; strengthens the legs; invokes a feeling of courage and fearlessness

Props: Yoga mat

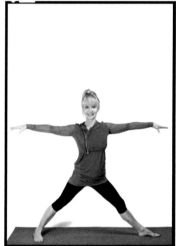

1. Stand in the mountain pose in the centre of your mat, so that the mat is oriented width ways.
2. Stand with your feet wide and open your arms out to the sides. Your feet should be aligned just below your wrists. Make sure that your feet are parallel. Spread your toes and root down through the four corners of your feet.
3. Turn your left foot in slightly and turn the right foot directly out to the side. Line up your right foot with the middle of the arch of your left foot.
4. Gently firm your leg muscles. Rotate your right thigh outwards so that the knee lines up with the foot. Turn the ribcage to face front as in the mountain pose.
5. Softly draw your tailbone down, relax your shoulders and extend up through the crown of the head (picture a string pulling you up from the crown of your head). Stretch out through your fingertips.

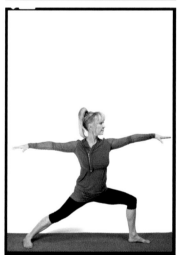

6. Inhale. On the exhale, bend the right knee to a 90° angle. Strongly ground your back leg. Keep the front knee in line with the foot and over the ankle.
7. Look out over your front hand. Relax your eyes and extend out in a direct line from the heart through the fingertips. Invoke the inner stance of a warrior.
8. Take five smooth, steady breaths and on an inhale, straighten your front leg, turn your feet to face forward and step the feet back together, releasing your arms down by your sides. Repeat on the other side.

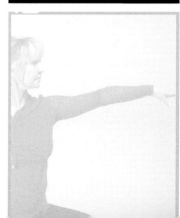

WIDE-LEGGED STANDING FORWARD BEND

Benefits: **Calming; opens the hips; stretches the inner and back thighs; releases the neck**

Props: **Yoga mat**

1 Stand in the mountain pose in the centre of your mat, so that the mat is oriented width ways.

2 Stand with your feet wide apart and open your arms out to the sides. Your feet should be aligned with your wrists. Make sure your feet are parallel. Spread your toes and root down through the four corners of the feet, firming the entire leg.

3 Place your hands on your hips.

4 Inhale, open the chest and look upwards. On the exhale, bend forward at the hips and place your fingertips on the floor below your shoulders. (Bend your knees if you can't reach the floor.)

5 Keeping the legs strong, softly stretch the chest forwards and look forwards.

6 On an exhale, walk your hands back in line with your feet and release your torso and head down towards the floor.

7 Continue to keep your legs firm, while allowing your spine to completely release. At the same time, draw your shoulder blades towards your waist and fully release your neck.

8 Breathe softly along the spine.

9 On an inhale, root your feet and walk your hands forwards. Bend your knees, place your hands on your hips and, leading with your heart, come up. Step the feet together and stand in the mountain pose.

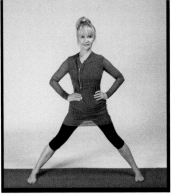

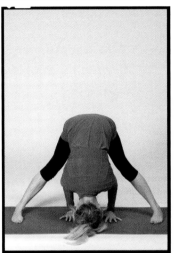

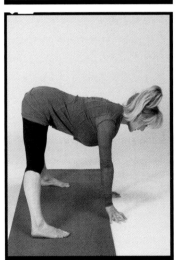

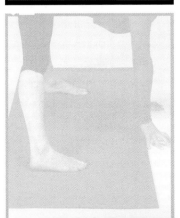

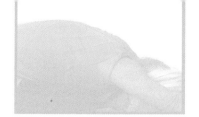

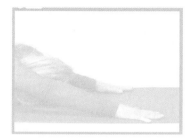

EASY SITTING POSE STRETCHING FORWARDS

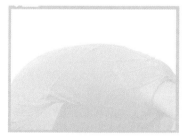

Benefits: **Calming; opens the hips; gently stretches the back**

Props: **Yoga mat and blanket**

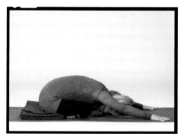

1   Sit cross-legged on a blanket on top of your mat.
2   Place your feet directly below your knees so that your shins are crossed and rest on the outer edges of your feet. Place your fingertips on the mat by your hips.
3   Pressing down through your fingertips, softly roll your shoulders back and lengthen your trunk so that you are sitting right up on your buttocks.

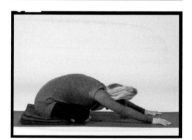

4   Release your knees down and soften your hips.
5   Inhale. On the exhale, begin to walk your hands forward. As you do so, root back through your hips.
6   Softly release the back of your neck and head downwards.
7   Imagine that you are breathing into your back and breathing into your hips.

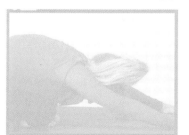

8   On an inhale, walk your hands back and come up.
9   Change the crossing of your legs (so that if your left leg was on top, switch so that your right leg is now on top), and repeat on the other side.

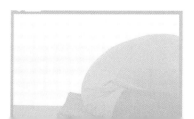

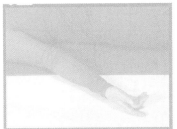

CORPSE POSE
(ten to fifteen minutes)

Benefits: **Calming and rejuvenating; a complete relaxation of the body; centring; quiets the mind; deepens the breath**

Props: **Yoga mat and blanket**

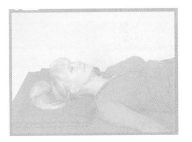

1 Lie on your back with your knees bent. Place the folded blanket underneath your neck and head.

2 Adjust your shoulder blades down your back, so that your shoulders soften and move back towards the floor and your chest broadens and lifts.

3 Push the flesh of your buttocks down towards your heels to lengthen the lower back.

4 Release your legs down to the floor and place your arms slightly away from the body, palms up.

5 Close your eyes and begin to pay attention to your breath. With each exhale, allow the body to completely relax.

6 Let the back of the body broaden into the floor as if you were melting.

7 Keep your mind centred in your breath.

8 Cultivate evenness in your breathing while completely relaxing the breathing.

9 Relax the muscles of your eyes, tongue and lips. Completely relax the skin of your forehead and soften your brow.

10 In this way, allow yourself to completely relax.

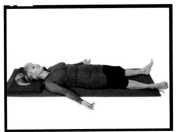

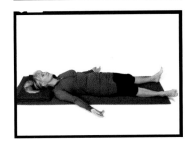

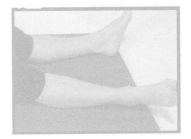

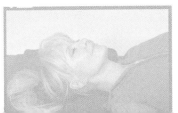

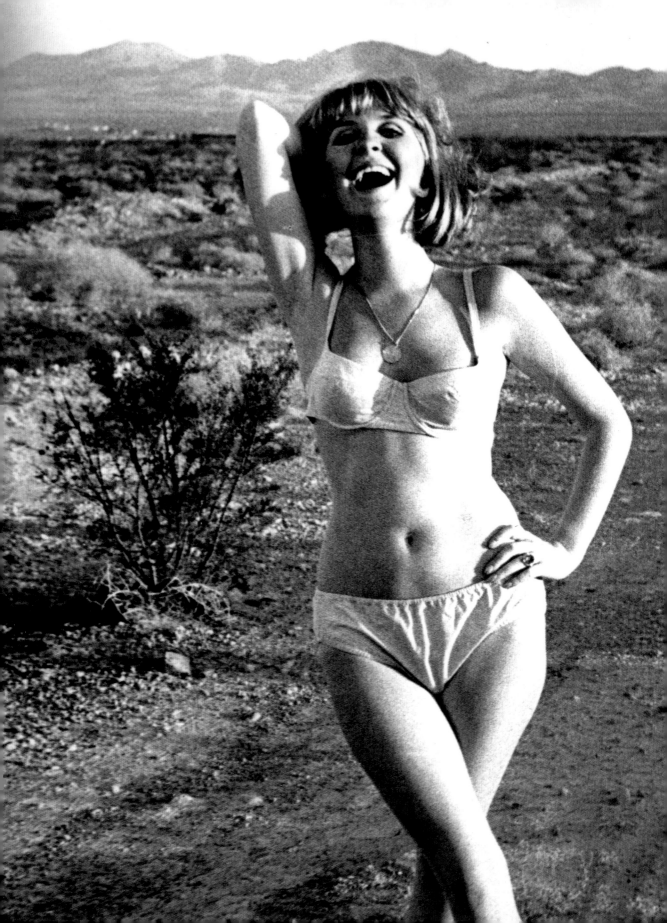

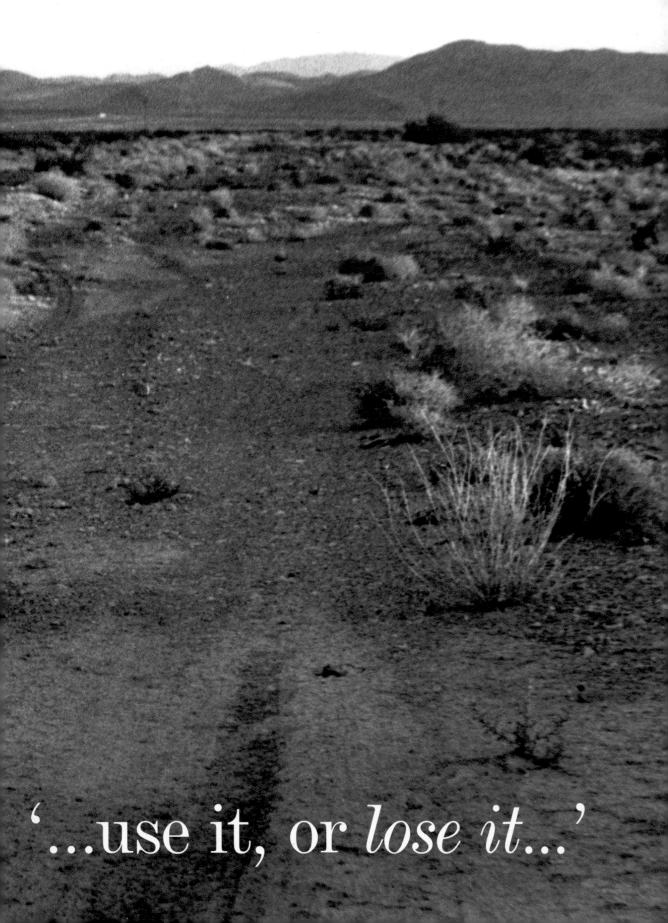

'...use it, or *lose it*...'

Walk On By

I used to be a runner. I loved it — till my knees started to give out on me and, trust me, that's *not* fun. Actually, I was a late starter: I didn't start running until I was in my early forties. My son Jordan was at school in America and into track running, and he said, 'You know, Mum, I think you'd be good at running: you're very fit and agile.' I'd never run in my life. Not even for a bus! But within a year — at the time I was doing a demanding stage show with Take That — I was doing six miles, four or five days a week.

I was fantastically aerobically fit. I felt great. But I was running on tarmac and along the canal, all the way from Camden to Maida Vale and back, beating the

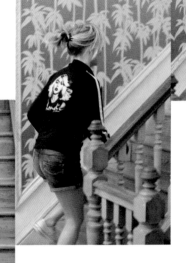

It's the little bits of exercise throughout the day that add up. Make it your priority to always take the stairs.

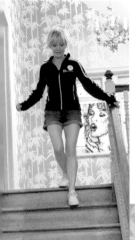

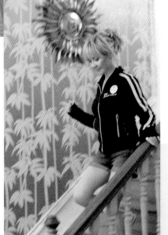

pavements. My knees weren't even cushioned by me running on grass — and that's tough for anyone over 40: you're just asking for joint problems, which is exactly what happened to me. Ouch. So now I walk. I take the dogs and I walk in the park, preferably on a soft surface, wearing cushioned shoes, which is w-a-y gentler on the joints. By the way, it helps if you can buddy up with a friend to go walking (unless you have a particularly fierce-looking dog!). Some women feel vulnerable walking on their own. I get together with my friend Joyce and we set off round the park, and we're chatting, and before we know it, two fantastic gossipy calorie-burning hours have passed and we're both late for what we're meant to be doing next.

But I don't have to wait until I've laced up my walking shoes and stepped into the fresh air to get little repeated bursts of exercise throughout the day. If it's a choice between the lift and a few flights of steps, I take the steps every time. I walk to appointments and leave the car at home. And at home, I run up the stairs: it's a joke among my friends that here I am, in my sixties, and still running up the stairs like a six-year-old! I *purposely* fight any couch potato tendencies by going to the loo upstairs so it makes me run up there! But you know what? I plan to be running up the stairs like a six-year-old when I'm 80! Because when it comes to your body, I truly believe it's a case of use it, or lose it...

Gym *Will* Fix It

... If you can bear it! And I've certainly found that I need to do at least one or two sessions a week in the gym to maintain optimum fitness. Earlier in my career, I was on stage every day — often performing several times a day — and my body was in great, effortless shape. But I'm not rushing around touring all the time nowadays, so I have to work a little at staying trim and toned. Frankly, for most women a combination of walking, with some gentle weights and stretching (preferably yoga-style) is all you need. I still have — still *want* — to get up on stage and skip around in leggings and tight pants. So I've got to go the extra distance with my trainer, Jon Goodair.

He gets me skipping sideways, forwards and backwards on the treadmill. At the beginning, I thought he was trying to kill me, but now I can do it for 10 minutes. (He'd like me to always do 20 minutes or more. Sometimes it's war!) Jon's point is that you have to challenge yourself, and that skipping in one direction wouldn't give the same all-over workout. I also do some hand weights. I asked Jon for some simple exercises that you can do at home, to get many of those same benefits.

It's hard. *Really* hard. But it's music that gets me through it — and what I know is that you can find the songs, the singers and the beat that will motivate you, too. The iPod is one of the greatest inventions *ever* — because it lets you put together your perfect playlists for your chosen exercise. You can have a walking workout playlist (start with some slower music, build up the pace and slow down again for a cool-down at the end), and a more pumpin', rockin' gym playlist that you can listen to on the treadmill, or while doing weights. There are even special

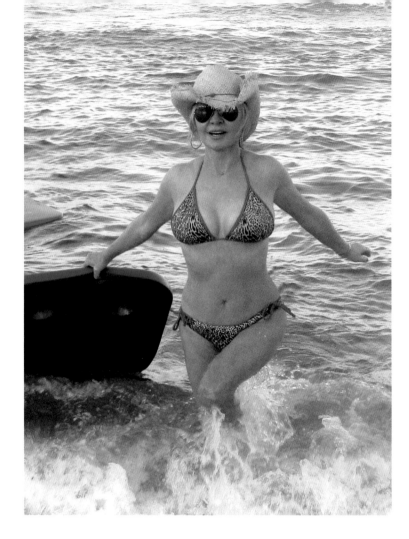

The paparazzi took this photo of me coming out of the sea on holiday. Working out makes me feel so much more confident in a bikini!

waterproof cases that will let you listen to your iPod as you do your laps in the pool. Handel's Water Music or The Beach Boys? The whole point is: *you* get to choose what's on that playlist. (I long to be able to swim better, by the way: I swim like the Loch Ness Monster with my neck sticking up out of the pool! My great friend Susannah Constantine — of Trinny and Susannah — and I are always going on about having swimming lessons so that we can power up and down the pool doing the crawl. And you know what? I *will* one of these days!)

Whatever exercise you're doing, though (unless it's a team sport), music just makes the time pass more quickly when you're working out: you can *lose* yourself in the music, and hey! Twenty minutes are up, just like that. And you've put a great big 'tick' in the box that says 'Exercise' on your To Do List. How great is that?

Dance, Little Lady, *Dance*

I *love* to dance. On stage, off stage, in my bedroom, at parties.
Of course I used to jive when I was younger. I remember many
years ago I went to a club with a whole load of actors, and we
salsa danced together — and I just got my feet trodden on all
night! Did I care? No, because I've always loved the idea of
dancing with a partner. Still, that bruised-toe episode made me
determined to learn to dance properly one day. So last year I did
exactly that and took up salsa. So romantic. So sensual. *So* good
for the hips and waist and thighs!

This is *not* something you're going to be able to learn at home
with a DVD, though. You need to sign up for lessons, at a dance
school, in a church hall — honestly, like yoga, there are classes
all over the place. And, as with just about any form of exercise,
it's great to go with a friend — for the laughter factor, when you
catch each other's eye across the room. Makes it more fun,
somehow, and a good laugh releases all the tension.

Maybe you don't want to learn salsa, but you rather like the idea
of line-dancing, or rock 'n' roll, or even (after all those Saturday
nights in front of *Strictly Come Dancing*) the foxtrot or the
quickstep. It doesn't matter. It gets you on your feet, gets your
heart pumping and fills you with pure, unadulterated joy when
you finally get a few steps right.

I was bursting with energy
when I first started in the music
business and I'm determined to
stay that way. I just have to
work at it a little harder now…

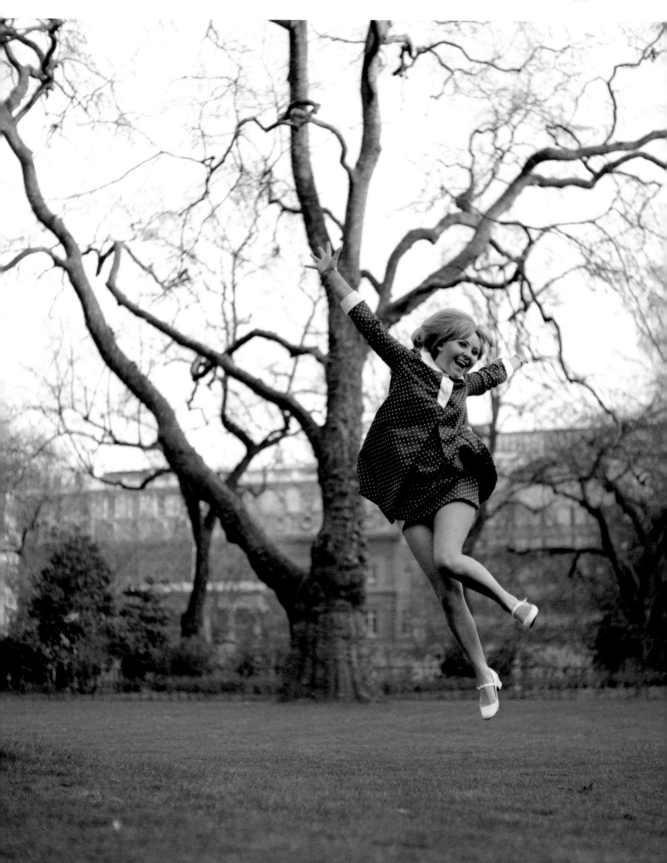

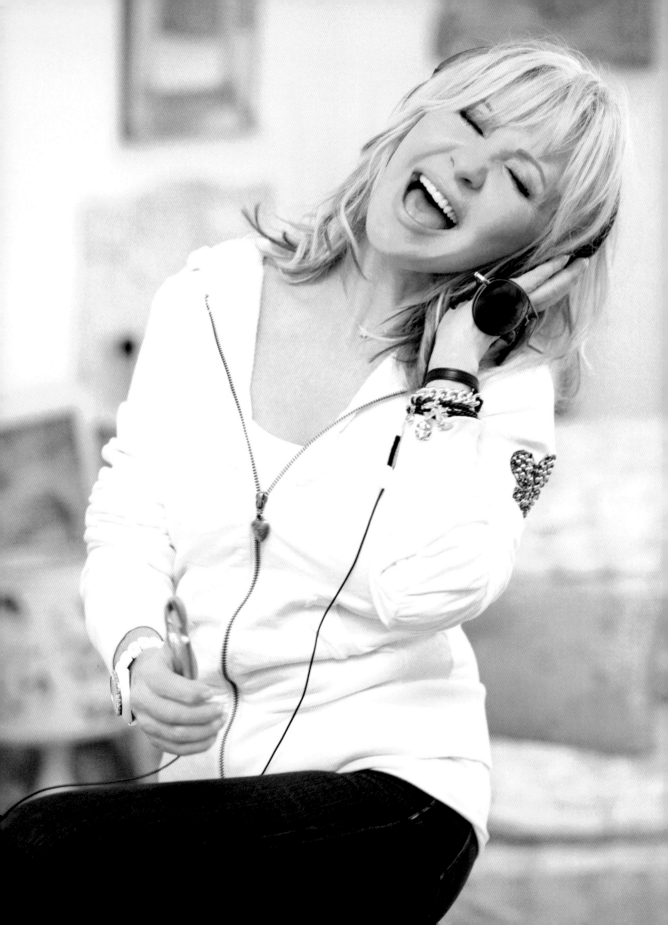

MUSIC WHILE YOU WORK (OUT).....

When I go to the gym, I work out to these...

- 'B in the Mix' (The Remixes) — Britney Spears
- 'Forever' — Chris Brown
- 'Good Girl Gone Bad' (The Remixes) — Rihanna
- 'Timbaland Presents Shock Value' — Timbaland
- 'Poker Face' — Lady Gaga
- 'Will.i.am' — will.i.am
- 'Kylie X' — Kylie Minogue
- 'The Duchess' — Fergie
- 'Blackout' — Britney Spears
- 'Year of the Gentleman' — Ne-yo
- 'Just Dance' — Lady Gaga

Salsa Your Way Slim

My salsa classes actually inspired me to take my dancing a stage further: some American girlfriends and I booked in for 'Dance Week' at the Canyon Ranch Spa in the US. We did four or five hours of dance a day, which was completely fabulous — a total treat, even though I fell into bed utterly exhausted at the end of the day, and slept like a baby. I'm not a ballet person, so I did hip-hop. I had a Michael Jackson class, rock and jazz — and at the end of it we learned a piece to perform (which, let me tell you, even for someone who's used to getting up on stage was a pretty scary thing!). But, as vacations go, it beat lying on a beach hands down. Action. Fun. Movement. Loads and loads and loads of laughter. And thousands of calories burned! I plan to do it every year from now on.

If you think about it, there's probably an all-action, keep-you-fit holiday you'd enjoy, too, which will enhance and build your fitness much better than lounging on a recliner drinking Piña Coladas. (Though we all have to do that, from time to time.) Just remember to pack your dancing shoes!

Music is my passion and nothing fails to improve my mood and energize me like my favourite songs.

Worth the *Weights*

It isn't just muscles that we need to keep strong as we get that bit older: it's bones. Of course, if you work a muscle, you see the results very quickly. The effect that exercise has on bones is invisible — but it's soooooooooooo important, in order to help prevent osteoporosis.

I know that yoga can help strengthen bones in the upper body because you're putting your weight on your hands, shoulders and spine, and it's weight-bearing exercise that does that particular trick. (Swimming, unfortunately, doesn't work in the same way because we weigh so much less in the water, so there's less resistance, and you don't get the same bone-building effect.) But doing some gentle work with weights or stretchy bands at home is like an insurance policy against osteoporosis. I'm the first to admit, though, that I'm no pro when it comes to telling anyone how and what they should be lifting weight-wise, so I asked my trainer Jon Goodair for some simple moves that just about anyone can do.

I try to visit Jon — who set up and runs the wonderful gym at Home House, in London — at least twice a week, for cardio and resistance work. So I asked him to explain some of the exercises he gets me to do...

Jon puts the emphasis on keeping the workout varied — mixing it up, the way I like it. If you're doing different movements, it's less boring and your co-ordination improves enormously.

JON'S BASIC RULES...

Resistance work
- Quality is better than quantity.
- Work S-L-O-W-L-Y and use breathing to control your speed.

Cardio
- Aim for 40 minutes of cardio at least 4 times per week.
- Vary the type of training you do, as well as the intensity and duration of each workout.
- Learn your heart rate training zones.

Stretching
- Hold a stretch for 15 seconds to one minute.
- Stretch all major muscle groups and never bounce a stretch.

Posture
- Where there is tightness: Stretch.
- Where there is shortness: Lengthen.
- Where there is weakness: Strengthen.

B-R-E-A-T-H-E...

The simple rule with all these exercises is: exhale when you're exerting yourself and inhale on the 'return' movement.

Cardio

ON-THE-SPOT SKIPPING

Skip twice on one leg, lifting the other leg slightly. Then switch. Switch back. (This is all pretty fast.) Skip forward for eight skips, then back for eight skips, and sideways, first one side, then the next. This is great for getting your heart pumping (though if you're not used to exercising, take it easy). Gradually, build up until you can do this for five to ten minutes.

ON THE REBOUND(ER)

I use the rebounder (like a mini-trampoline) at Home House; these are great because they're gentle on the knees. (They're not expensive so you might want to buy one for your home.) Put the music on and start moving around, gently jumping up and down on one or two feet. Move sideways a bit, forwards, backwards — and try little mini-jacks, lifting your arms up to shoulder level as you jump; the more variety the better. Again, start with a couple of minutes, then build up.

Resistance Work

Start with these exercises for a really good overall workout that will build strength and make your silhouette sleek – without bulking you up…

THE
DOOR-PULL

Take a stretchy rubber 'Dyna-Band' (see p.266) and hook it over
an immoveable coat hook — if you've got one on the back of the
bedroom or bathroom door, that's ideal. Take hold of the ends of
the band, one in each hand, and draw your arms backwards,
outwards and down — a slow rowing action. This will isolate the
'lats', or back muscles. Repeat ten times, very slowly. (As you
build up, you can do two or three sets). If you raise your arms to
shoulder level and do the same exercise, it's a great workout for
your shoulder muscles. (The wonderful thing about these rubber
bands is that they're ultra-light, so they're easy to pack when
you travel.)

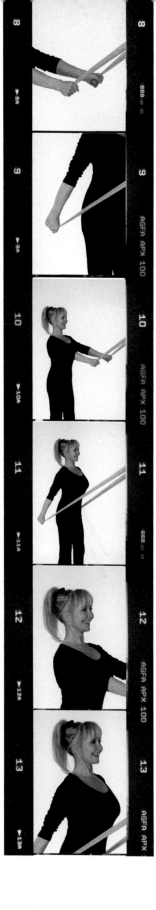

THE
MONKEY

You'll need 1.5 Kg/3 lb. weights for this (and the exercises that follow). I like the foam-covered ones that Jon uses, which are easy to hold. Stand with your feet hip-distance apart, weight evenly balanced between the balls of your feet and your heels. Engage the stabilising muscles in your inner thighs and pelvic floor. Bend your knees slightly, roll your shoulders back and open your collarbone. Hold one of the weights in one hand, at your side. Curl the arm up and lift the weight towards your armpit, trying not to lift your shoulder. Repeat eight times, then change arms. Build up to 16 reps on each side.

BICEP CURL
AND
PRESS

Do the same as above, but turn your hand so that your arm is in front of you and you are lifting the weight towards your shoulder, then overhead. Again, repeat eight to 16 times.

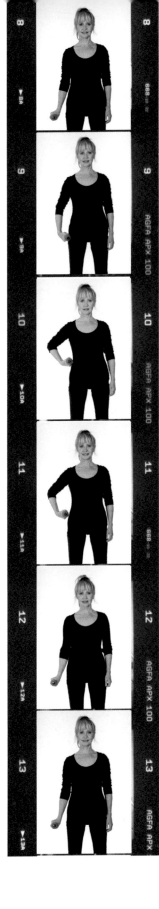

OVERHEAD
TRICEPS
EXTENSION

Take the weight in one hand. Here, one arm is raised up above
your head, shoulders relaxed. Drop the hand of your raised arm
behind you. (If you're a beginner and unused to weights, you can
use the other hand to support the raised arm. Or, to start with,
don't use weights at all, and rely on the weight of your own arm.
It'll still work.) When you've been doing this for a while, you can
do this on a big inflatable stability ball. (These are also great for
helping stability — just sitting on one and trying not to roll around
will help your all-important core muscles.) Roll your body down
the ball so that your legs are in front of you, feet below knees,
and you are resting back on the ball with your shoulders. Take
the weight in one hand and do your triceps curl in this position.

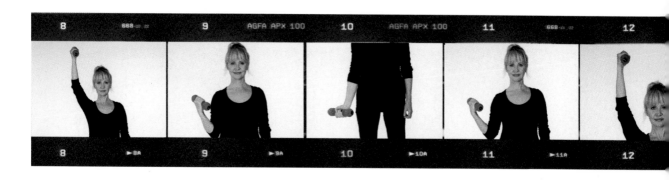

CHEST FLYES

This is another slightly more advanced exercise using the stability ball. In the same position as below, with shoulders resting on the ball and legs in front of you, knees bent, take one weight in each hand. Imagine you were holding a big ball — that's the shape you're trying to create with your arms. Keep your arms straight and lower them down in line with your shoulders to slightly above shoulder level.

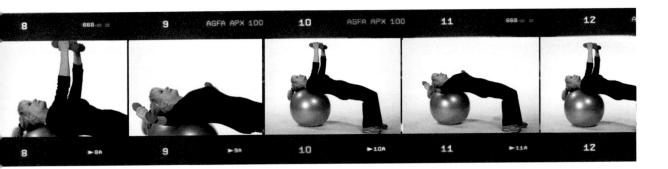

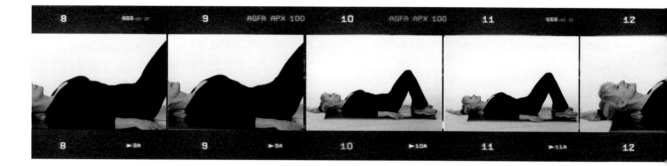

TUMMY FLATTENER

This is the one every woman wants! Lie on your back, with your knees bent at a 90° angle and your lower legs resting on a stool or a low chair, for support. Without gripping your buttocks, slowly pull your belly button towards your spine: imagine it being drawn down by an invisible hand. Slowly release. Repeat 10 times. Build up over time — this will help create a wonderful 'natural corset' of core abdominal muscles.

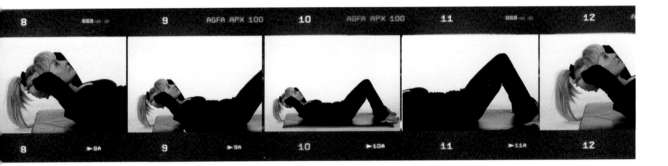

A KINDER KIND OF CRUNCH

Some abdominal crunches can strain the neck or back, and you absolutely want to avoid that. Stay in the same position as for Tummy Flattener. Cradle your head in your hands and gently — very gently — curl forward, keeping your neck as long as possible and not crunching it towards your chest. (Imagine you have a ripe peach under your chin, or put a squishy ball there.) Do not pull your elbows together when you lift your head, but try to engage the abdominal muscles. Start with a few, and you'll find you soon can build up.

OBLIQUE CRUNCH

Stay in the same position as before, but this time cradle your head in one hand, reaching the other arm straight behind you. Curl forward bringing the extended arm over, reaching the finger tips to the front of the opposite thigh.

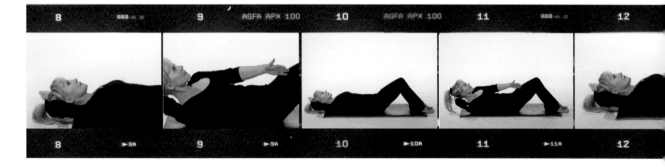

LEG LIFT

Lie on your back. Put your hands under the small of your back,
palms down, to offer a little extra lower back support. You
should feel the pressure on your fingers so that you know
you're maintaining your spine in the correct position. Bend your
legs at the knee, and slowly lift your leg until it's at a 90° angle
to the floor (engage the tummy muscles while you do this —
that's what you're after). Do ten on one side, then ten on the
other. Or do alternate legs for 20. Vary the number of reps
from workout to workout.

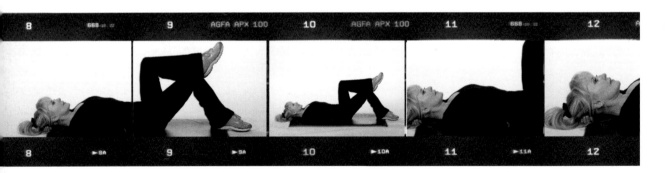

I've found out what works for me, but what works for you might be a bit different. The bottom line is: you have to get some aerobic exercise (at least three times a week for 20 minutes. They do say five times a week, but show me a woman who can manage that!), and do something that stretches out the muscles, at least several times a week but preferably every day. And that way – trust me – you can maintain that bombshell body for as long as you're prepared to work at it, even just a little.

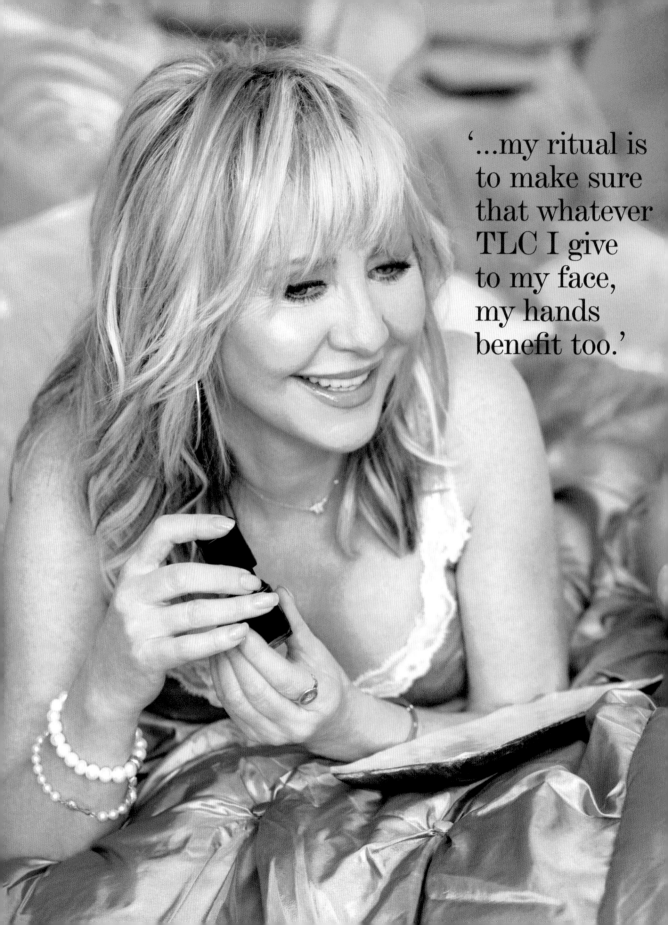

'...my ritual is to make sure that whatever TLC I give to my face, my hands benefit too.'

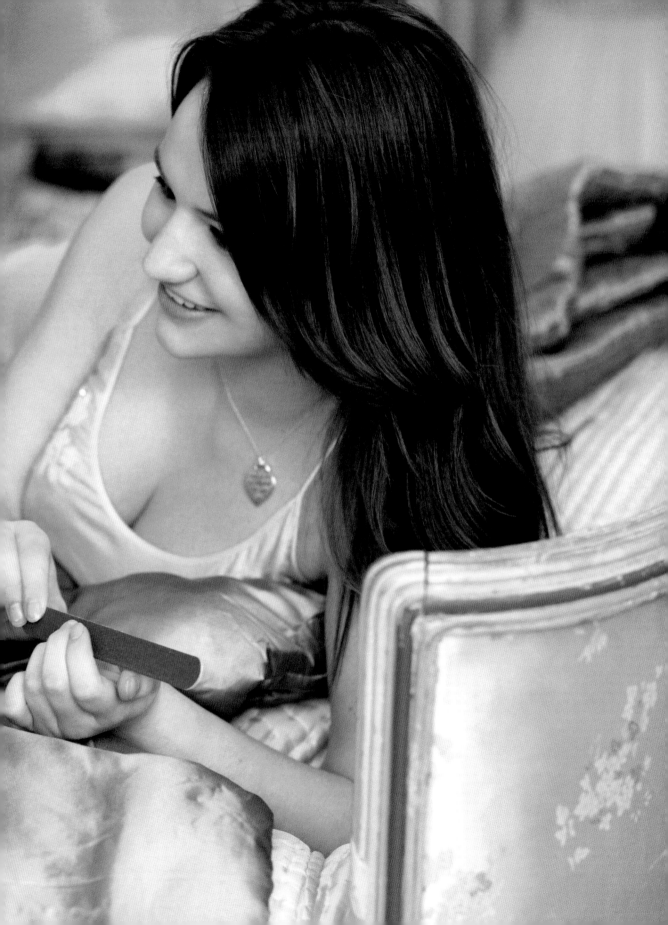

Hands *and* Feet

If you're working out, or walking, or generally taking care of your body, then it's nice to treat yourself to a little pampering, to reward yourself for those efforts.

I think it helps to think of caring for the hands and feet as an extension of facial care. Or at least it should be, because the skin on the hands and feet can look dry and papery, or younger and fresher (and I know which I prefer). So here are my thoughts on those 'extremities', our hands and feet, which work so hard for us and get so little attention...

Hands Up, Baby, Hands Up

Hands can be an instant age giveaway. Oh, yes. So my ritual is to make sure that whatever TLC I give to my face, my hands benefit, too. It's a golden rule for me: whatever I'm applying to my face, I use the 'leftovers' on my hands. Face cream, masks, my Youth Juice Oil. If there's so much as a smidgen left over, I smooth it into hands, and especially into my cuticles. I also keep hand cream by the sink (I've got my own hand cream now; it's called Hand to Hand Combat. But before that my favourite was Olivina Lavender Hand Cream, which smells of California to me — more like citrus than lavender). For me it's important that a cream is nourishing, yet sinks in pretty quickly.

But don't stop with hand cream... Any rich, emollient oil or cream can do the trick. If you're cooking, smooth some of the cooking oil into your hands. Or even butter! And if you're applying cream to a baby's skin, lavish some extra on your hands at the same time. It's the perfect way to keep them soft and smooth as — yes, a baby's bottom.

The tip when applying hand cream is not just to rub it between your palms, but to apply it carefully to the backs of your hands and down your arms as if you were pulling on a pair of tight gloves, really working it into the skin in smooth, gliding movements. Another good tip for cuticle care is to use a combination of argan oil and olive oil and rub into your cuticles for added moisture.

My nails are always manicured (although I get into trouble with my manicurist because I tend to open cans with my nails, and all the things that you're *not* meant to do if you want lovely nails). Manicures are a luxury I got into the habit of in the US, where there are $10 Korean manicurists on every corner — but even if you can't afford a regular manicure, then I think it is a sign of self-esteem to make sure nails are perfectly groomed, and to do them regularly yourself. (So over the page you'll see an easy how-to for a home manicure.)

Personally, I like deep polish shades for winter, like Essie Material Girl (an ultra-deep burgundy), and either a hot pink or a French manicure for summer. When I see strangers checking me out, they always look me up and down and check out my nails — so I make sure I'm not going to give them the satisfaction of catching me with chipped nail polish! And why should you be any different?

'HANDS CAN BE AN INSTANT AGE GIVEAWAY.'

What you need for the perfect manicure:

Hand and cuticle cream
Nail oil
Buffer
Soft grade natural nail file
Rubber hoof stick
Nail clippers
Base and top coats
Nail polish
Nail polish remover
Cotton pads
Nail quick-dry

* Remove any old polish by soaking a cotton pad in nail-polish remover and holding onto the nail for a few seconds, then wiping away.

* File nails using a gentle, cushioned nail file (never metal). Always file in one direction only; if you use a sawing motion, you lift the nail layers away from each other. (If you must clip your nails first because they're way too long, then do so.)

* Gently buff nails with a buffer to enhance shine (and boost blood flow, bringing nutrients to the nail); you should never do this so hard or for so long that the nails start to warm up, though. Lightly does it.

* Push back the cuticles with a hoof stick. Don't cut the cuticles, ever — and I advise never allow them to be cut in a nail salon, either; the more you cut, the more they grow.

✳ If nails are stained, rub with a grapefruit skin or the inside of a lemon peel to lift the colour. (Half a lemon is great for rubbing on dry elbows, too — Barbara Streisand used to swear by that trick!)

✳ Apply a base coat to smooth out nail ridges and allow to dry for two minutes, minimum.

✳ Paint on the first coat of colour, and then wait for two minutes. (If you smudge onto the skin around the nails, lift the polish off with the tip of an orange stick.) Apply a second coat, and again wait for two minutes. The time you spend waiting for the nails to dry properly between coats is an investment: the longer you wait, the longer your manicure will last.

✳ Apply a top coat, either a quick-drying product or, if you've got the leisure time to languish while you allow your nails to dry, then apply a regular top coat and r-e-l-a-x.

✳ Add a few drops of nail quick-dry after a minute or two. If you've got to run out the door, add a drop or two of oil to each nail. This will prevent fluff sticking to the surface and does double-duty by helping to 'set' the polish.

Hands need sun protection, too, because they're just as vulnerable as your face. Keep a tube of sun cream in the car (or in your handbag), and apply it to the backs of your hands, wrists and forearms when you're about to get out of the car on a sunny day, to shield them from damage.

Feet, Don't Fail Me Now

I would say to every single woman out there: even if you can't afford the luxury of a regular pedicure, book in for one, once a year — preferably at the start of summer, to prep your feet for sandal season and the beach. The point is once a professional's done the serious 'footwork', it's easy to maintain feet at home. If you have problems like bunions or corns, see a chiropodist or a podiatrist. (I had a little bunion, from all those years of squeezing my feet into pointy shoes.) Foot problems have a major impact on the rest of the body: if your feet hurt, you won't walk; if you don't walk, your weight may creep up — and so it goes on... My feet *have* to be happy.

The key to a fabulous home pedicure — to keep up that good work — is to arrange all your supplies around you, and then follow these instructions step–by–step.

Soak
Fill a deep bowl with warm water and add a foot soak, or even just a few drops of peppermint essential oil. You can add a pint of milk or a cupful of dried milk powder, to make the water super-softening. Before you soak, remove nail polish (if any), saturating the cotton pads in nail-polish remover, pressing on to the nail for a few minutes and then wiping off. Immerse your feet for two to three minutes, then dry with a towel.

File
File toenails straight across to avoid ingrown nails. Leave around one-eighth of an inch showing. (If nails are long, clip them first — but be careful not to cut right down to the quick.)

Give your cuticles some TLC

Apply cuticle oil or remover and massage for a minute or two. Push cuticles back with a rubber hoof stick. (Metal or wood implements may nick them, which is risky because the cuticle is a natural barrier to keep bacteria from entering your body.)

Buff

Even an expensive sandal looks like it cost £5 if you have dry heels! (I see all sorts of feet at my yoga classes and I am often amazed at how dry women's heels and soles are.) Slough off dead skin from the heel, arch, ball, ankle and toes with a foot buffer or a salt or sugar scrub — but use a light touch: if you rub too hard, you actually compact the layers of skin, creating calluses rather than eliminating them. (The Alida Foot File is amazing: it looks like a cheese grater, but it gently buffs feet until they're super-smooth with no risk of cutting or nicking.)

Slather

Take time to massage a rich cream into your feet — but avoid getting lotion between your toes, as moisture in that area may apparently lead to fungal conditions like athlete's foot. After you've rubbed in the cream, wrap your feet in dry towels and let them sit for five minutes; your body heat will warm up the moisturiser and help it really sink in.

Clean

Wash your feet thoroughly with a liquid soap wash and use a nailbrush to get under the nails.

Polish

Thoroughly wipe your toenails and cuticles with a cotton ball soaked in nail-polish remover (oil or moisturiser prevents polish from going on evenly). Paint nails with a basecoat, two coats of colour and a top coat.

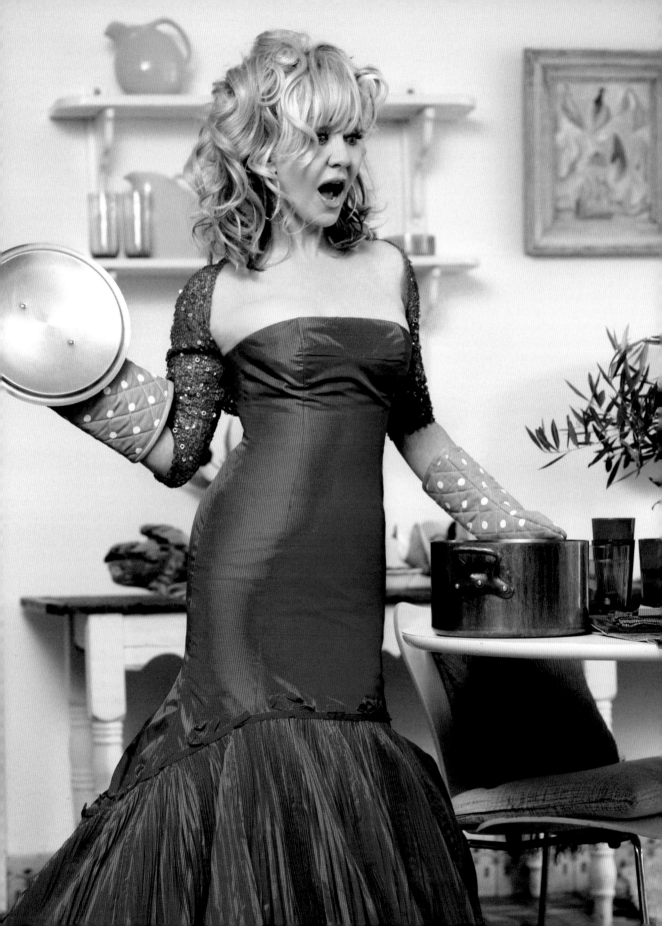

Food For Thought

For the Love of *Food*

As a child, I was always hungry — and it's not like my parents didn't feed me! My dad was a butcher and would bring home amazing cuts of meat, and he'd do a swap with the fishmongers so he'd get terrific fish, too. But I used to be able to eat what was on my plate, and half of what was left on everyone else's, and still I'd feel hungry. Maybe there was an emotional factor: my mum sometimes worked, so often I'd come home to an empty house and make myself a bowl of Bird's custard. Total comfort food. My mum would get home and say, 'Where's that pint of milk I bought?', and I'd have to tell her I'd made it into custard. Glasgow, of course, is famous as the homeland of the deep-fried Mars Bar. Now, I've never had one of those — ours was a Blue Riband house, actually (do you remember those chocolate-covered wafers?) — but I am a sugar addict, with a fairly typical Scottish hunger for sweets. So let me tell you how I've worked to conquer that, over the years.

'WE ARE WHAT WE REPEATEDLY DO. EXCELLENCE, THEN, IS NOT AN ACT, BUT A HABIT.'

Aristotle

The food I eat now is quite different to the food that I was raised on, you see. But over the years I've learned what works best for me and my metabolism. I was never overweight when I was young (despite all that custard), because I was so naturally active (some would say *hyper*active!) and physical. Then I got into the music business and started spending my life in the back of a van, belting from venue to venue and eating mostly at motorway caffs and roadside diners. I could have written a guide to the service stations of the M1, or got a degree in Little Chefs! There I was, surrounded by six men — all Glaswegians, except the roadie — stopping off for a fry-up, a curry or a Chinese after the show, with steak and kidney pie for breakfast and chocolate virtually round-the-clock, just to keep us going. I even took up smoking because I thought it would help me lose weight — but it didn't!

I really wanted to be skinny, because I was friendly with all those great beauties like Patti Boyd and Jean Shrimpton, Britt Ekland and Julie Christie, who were basically stick insects with lollipop legs. I was *way* shorter than anyone else (but I made more noise, to make up for it!). Which is how I started to do just about every diet known to woman. Unlike some girls I knew, I could never reel off the calorific value of everything from a Twix to an apple or a knob of cheese, but I've 'F-Planned'. I've food-combined. (Actually, what I eat now still incorporates some elements of food combining, so that definitely works for me.) I was a vegetarian for a while. I even invented my very own patented 'Coffee Diet', which was exclusive to me: I lived on coffee and I'd be shaking and almost insane by teatime and have to have chocolate in my mouth. Because, of course, the minute you start to deprive yourself... ALL YOU CAN THINK ABOUT IS FOOD! So that's how I learned that there had to be a better way. And what I realised is that dieting doesn't work. What you've got to do is change your eating habits.

Get food
Fabulous!

Beating the Sugar Blues

When I first arrived in London, I used to hang out in health-food shops, because I was interested in learning about healthy eating and I figured that was the best way to learn. And I picked up some books by a famous American nutritionist called Gayelord Hauser, who was dead set against sugar (and in favour of foods like whole grains). I bought books like *Look Younger; Live Longer*, *Be Happier, Be Healthier* and *Diet Does It*, and they inspired me to start to eat more healthily and learn to beat my sugar addiction. Gayelord Hauser was this glamorous Hollywood diet guru whose devotees included movie stars like Paulette Goddard, Greta Garbo, Marlene Dietrich — and, later, Grace Kelly and the Duchess of Windsor. Gloria Swanson — the fabulous star of films like *Sunset Boulevard* — was another HUGE heroine of mine, whose autobiography I just devoured. She insisted she'd cured herself of cancer by sunbathing (not sure about that, but it was a great read), and she was big on detoxing when nobody even knew what the word meant. In her book, glamorous Gloria talked a lot about diet — and, in fact, her sixth (yes, *sixth*!) husband was the bestselling author of *Sugar Blues*, which also ranted against sugar. Through those books, I learned that I was a sugar addict. And not, at that stage, a recovering one!

'FOR ME, BEING STOCKED UP WITH THE *RIGHT* FOOD HELPS.'

So I've learned that the main thing, for me, has been to stabilise my blood sugar — and I think that's true for so many people. Of course, there's virtually an epidemic of diabetes now, but many, many non-diabetics have blood sugar issues. If I don't eat regularly, I get wobbly and faint — and then I hit the chocolate, which is a disaster. So I know I have a tendency towards hypoglycaemia, and I need to listen to my body when it's telling me it needs fuel to bring it back into balance. Because I understand that about my body, in my fridge and my store cupboard I keep a supply of healthy snacks which aren't going to pile on the pounds, but will keep my blood sugar steady and my appetite in check. And that really *is* the key. If I ignore that shakiness, first of all I stop being able to think clearly. And then I literally start to wobble, both physically and emotionally, a wee bit, too. Before I know it, I'm completely ravenous and I'll eat everything in sight.

It is far better, then, to nip that tendency in the bud by having the right foods around me, on standby. It's a simple philosophy: if I eat something good, it'll stop me eating something bad. Because if you fill your fridge and cupboards with good foods — rather than junk — then it's so much easier to stay on the straight and narrow. If you're surrounded by sweet things, and you grab *those* when you've got the low blood sugar blues, the sweeties will send your blood sugar skyrocketing again — and dump you right down once more. Instead of being on a rollercoaster, think of it as being on a seesaw, and trying to stay near the middle, keeping your balance. For me, being stocked up with the *right* food helps.

My Breakfast

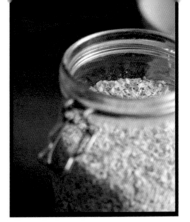

I start the day religiously with hot water and lemon juice. And then I have a slice of wholemeal sourdough toast with a scraping — and I mean a scraping — of goat's butter (tastes better than it sounds, and much better for the digestion than cow's butter), and hummus on top. If it's cold outside, then it's porridge season — like the good wee Scots lass I still am! (I add a swirl of agave syrup on top instead of sugar, and a splash of oat milk.) On the weekends it's *definitely* eggs — but during the week, too, I might have a boiled egg or two: hot and with a runny yolk, or hard-boiled and cold. Not every day, but once you tune into your body by starting to get off that sugar rollercoaster, it's so much easier to listen to what your body actually *needs*. My guilty secret? I have one nice big cup of *espresso*. I know I shouldn't, but it's part of my wake-up ritual — and it's the first *and* the last cup of coffee I'll have all day.

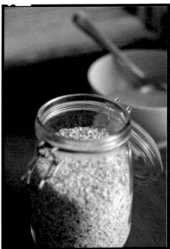

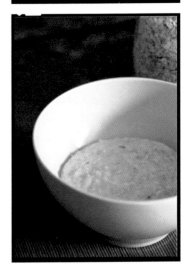

Porridge oats give slow-release energy and are the perfect breakfast choice at the start of a long day.

My Lunch

A portion of grilled or steamed fish or grilled/roast chicken — and I also love turkey burgers! Then, on the side, plenty of steamed vegetables, and probably a spoonful of *salsa*, too, to spice it all up. Or I might have some baked sweet potato, mashed with the skin on (the skin's packed with goodness). There's always a salad — although I'm Little Miss Fussy when it comes to salad — maybe some rocket and a mixture of lettuce, perhaps a few spinach leaves and some chicory or *radicchio* — but no tomatoes in the salad. (It's different if I'm going to a good Italian restaurant, where I LOVE a crunchy, fresh tomato-only salad, because they know where to source the best and most tomato-tasting tomatoes.)

My Dinner

This is pretty similar to lunch — the same but different, of course, because to be satisfied you've got to have variety. It's a fact: if you eat the same thing all the time out of habit, the appetite centre in the brain just doesn't register that you've eaten — so it's important to keep your palate excited. Supper's got to be really tasty, so I have a stash of cookbooks that tend to be the inspiration for my dinner, like *River Café Easy* by Rose Grey and Ruth Rogers, or Jamie Oliver's cookbooks. I love his Malaysian salad, or green beans and mustard, or the River Café's Swiss chard with chilli and garlic, or roast courgettes. I've trained my palate and my body to expect veg at every meal, and if I haven't, then I start craving them. So I often start with a bowl of my green soup, and then I'm really in heaven. Mmmmmmmmm.

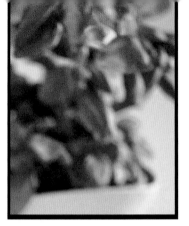

Lulu's Green Soup

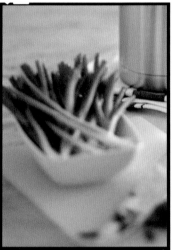

This green soup is great for using up veg that you've got in the fridge, so there's no waste. My son Jordan is a cook and he makes me up bags of chicken stock to use as a base for this — although Marigold Bouillon powder is also a great standby (Delia Smith swears by it...).

Basically, you add to the soup whatever is to hand: cabbage, cauliflower, spring onions, courgettes, peas, even lettuce — so long as it's green. Add these to the stock, boil until the vegetables are soft, and season to taste (lots of black pepper is *FABULOUS*!). You can then whizz it through the blender. If you prefer bigger chunks of vegetable, chop them to your preferred size before you put them into the stock. And I always add my big handful of chopped herbs on top.

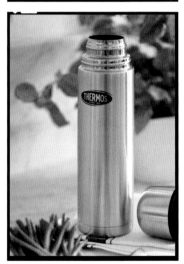

Invest in some small flasks for taking food-to-go with you. If you've got some hot, healthy soup in a flask, it helps you to resist the endless fast-food options — which are almost invariably high in fat and loaded with sugar.

My green soup is the ideal 'between-meals' healthy filler to keep me going without reaching for the biscuits.

The River Café's Braised Swiss Chard with Chilli and Garlic

Ruby chard and Bright Lights have tougher stalks than Swiss chard. Cut these off about five centimetres from the base of the leaf. Swiss chard in the summer has broader, more tender stalks and they are good to eat if they are white and crisp. If still green, cut them off as with the coloured chard. Cut the white stalks into one-centimetre slices.

Bring a large saucepan of salted water to the boil. If you have them, cook the stalks first for eight minutes. Remove with a slotted spoon. Cook the remaining leaves — you may have to do this in batches — for five minutes or until tender but still a little *al dente*. Drain and cool.

Heat the ghee in a very large, thick-bottomed frying pan. Add the garlic and cook briefly to soften it and flavour the oil, then add the crumbled chilli, fennel herb and the chard leaves and stalks. Stir them around in the pan to collect the flavours, then season generously. Serve with lemon wedges.

Vegetarian

For 6

500 g Swiss chard

500 g ruby chard

500 g Bright Lights chard

6 tablespoons ghee

6 garlic cloves, peeled and finely sliced

3 small dried red chillies, crumbled

2 tablespoons chopped fresh fennel herb

Maldon Salt and freshly ground black pepper

3 lemons, cut into wedges

Breaking Bad Habits

What I would say, though, is not to give yourself a hard time if you 'fall off the wagon', as it were, and have a binge. You *are* human. Be *kind* to yourself, rather than feel self-critical. I can't put my hand on my heart and say that eating healthily came naturally to me, or quickly. It's about vigilance. You've got to do it for long enough that it becomes a true habit. I'd love to wave my magic wand and promise overnight miracles, but life's not like that! Whatever you do, don't throw the baby out with the bathwater: if you eat too much sugar or fatty foods one day, don't think that's it; you're a failure, it's all over, so might as well give up. Nobody's perfect.

Remember:
tomorrow is another day. The next meal is a fresh start, and you can eat healthily then. (And if you're really, really having problems, it might help to join an organisation like Weight Watchers. I know people who've lost weight — and kept it off — by going to Weight Watchers. It's all about finding what works for you, and if you're better with the support of other people, it's an organisation that's worth checking out.)

I tell myself that nothing is forbidden. Yes, I weaned myself off having sugar in my tea (thanks to Gayelord and Gloria), but I didn't ban biscuits, for instance, because if someone told me I couldn't have a biscuit, all I'd think about was BISCUITS!

'IT DOES NOT MATTER HOW SLOWLY YOU GO, SO LONG AS YOU DO NOT STOP.'
Confucius

ZZZZZZZZ...

Want to know one of the most important lessons I've learned about weight loss? I try not to get tired. If I'm exhausted, I eat to give myself energy, and that's fatal. So one key tip is: a catnap or 20 minutes of meditation is better than a snack. (For more on SLEEP, see pp.242–3.)

It is really important to me to buy good, fresh, high-quality foods. Invest in quality, not quantity. Don't buy two-for-ones at the supermarket — because the temptation is just to eat more!

Chocolate is my comfort food nowadays, not custard. But, you know what? I've trained myself not to go there, by not having it in the house. If it's not there, I can't eat it. Growing up in a Blue Riband household, as I said, means now that crunchy, biscuity things are my weakness.

I sort of developed my own version of food combining, which really boiled down to not eating protein and carbohydrates at the same meal. Now — particularly in winter — I notice that my metabolism shifts again. I'll have a little mashed sweet potato with lunch or dinner, and if I have my nephews over, I'll mash new potatoes with some very finely chopped onions, which I've fried in canola oil until they're soft. But what I absolutely do *not* do, still, is eat potatoes with lashings of butter. It's actually far tastier just to add a twist of black pepper and a little drizzle of good organic extra virgin olive oil.

Here's what's changed about me over the years. Once upon a time I'd eat the whole packet of nuts, or a giant baked potato with lashings of butter, and maybe a second baked potato... And now I don't. I've trained myself. I didn't force it. It happened when I was in my late thirties, and I just began to change my habits. You can't force it, but you can keep coming back. But you know what? Having said all that, sometimes I just dig in and fill my face with a big bowl of pasta. The key is not to think you've blown it, that it's all over, if you do that. Like I say, it's all about vigilance, and eventually, the good habits start to become a way of life. It's about finding the discipline — but always dealing with yourself in a gentle and loving way.

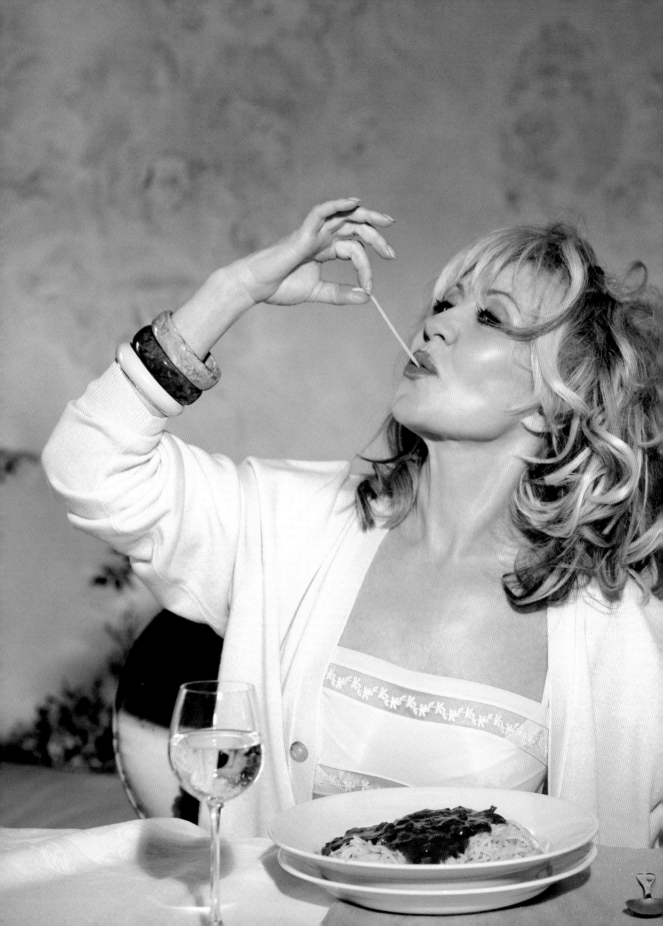

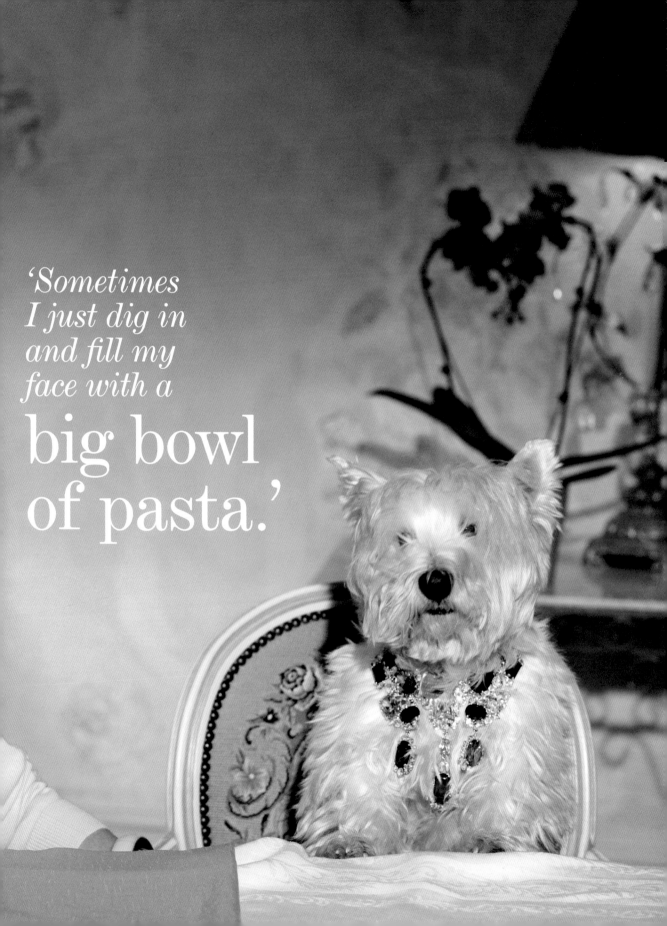

'Sometimes I just dig in and fill my face with a **big bowl of pasta.**'

Snack *Attacks*

This is what you'll find in my pantry and my fridge. I absolutely try not to eat between meals. But, for instance, I never eat immediately before I go on stage, so when I get home, I really need something.

So, if I'm hungry I might have a piece of toast and hummus, or a cracker and hummus or an avocado. (If you keep the bread in the freezer, sliced, you can defrost a slice at a time, which means that reaching for another slice becomes a conscious decision, rather than something you do on automatic pilot.) Or I might go for a handful of nuts. What I know now about nuts is that they are full of essential fatty acids (which are also brilliant for keeping skin lubricated from within). Or a couple of wafer-thin slices of ham with mustard to give it a kick. But NOT a biscuit! NOT a chocolate bar! Otherwise I'd be back on that rollercoaster before you can say 'Alton Towers'...

MY SNACK LIST...

- A jar of almonds
- A jar of walnuts
- Clearspring teriyake crackers
- Hummus
- Olives
- Thin-sliced ham (my favourite is from Wholefoods Market, and it's paper-thin)
- Wholemeal sourdough bread (Judges Bakery)
- A jar of pesto
- A homemade jar of the River Café's Salsa Rossa (see recipe p.172)
- A homemade jar of the River Café's Salsa Verde (see recipe p.173)
- Chopped fresh vegetable crudites (carrot sticks, cauliflower, broccoli, etc.). Marks & Spencer sell these (and I pick up quite a few snacks there)
- Avocados — to me they have all the comfort factor of custard: delicious as a snack with a splash of balsamic vinegar.

Lulu's Salad Dressing

In a screw-top jam jar, pour one measure of good quality vinegar to two measures of olive oil. (If you're using a good quality balsamic vinegar, you don't need as much as it's quite powerful.) Add a crushed clove of garlic, a smidgen of salt and pepper and a teaspoon or so of mustard. Then shake it up, baby! It's delicious. Try adding a little chopped-up chilli pepper if you want to spice it up, or try lemon juice instead of vinegar. Once you've got the basic proportions right, it's fun to experiment. And there's no 'hidden sugar' in this recipe, unlike so many shop-bought salad dressings.

Good quality balsamic vinegar

Good quality olive oil

1 garlic clove, peeled and crushed

Maldon Salt and freshly ground black pepper

1 teaspoon mustard, or to taste

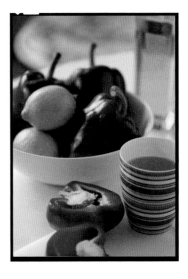

Salsa *Rossa*

Red Sauce. This is my equivalent of ketchup nowadays, which, as a child, I used to pour over just about everything I ate!

Peel and seed the peppers, then chop the flesh finely.

Heat the olive oil in a saucepan and gently fry the garlic until it starts to colour. Add the chilli and whole marjoram leaves and tomatoes and cook for thirty minutes or until the tomatoes are reduced. Add the peppers and cook for a further ten minutes. Season with salt and pepper and dried chilli.

Vegetarian

2 red peppers, grilled

2 tablespoons olive oil

1 garlic clove, peeled and finely chopped

1 fresh red chilli, seeded and finely chopped

1 tablespoon fresh marjoram leaves

4 ripe fresh tomatoes, skinned, or 1 x 250 g (8 oz) tin plum tomatoes, drained of their juices

Maldon Salt and freshly ground black pepper

2 small dried red chillies, crumbled

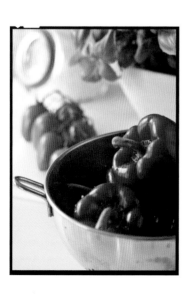

Salsa *Verde*

Green Sauce. Also extremely delicious and a useful sauce to add to just about anything.

If using a food processor, pulse-chop the parsley, basil, mint, garlic, capers and anchovies until roughly blended. Transfer to a large bowl and add the vinegar. Slowly pour in the olive oil, stirring constantly until combined, and finally add the mustard and stir. Check for seasoning.

This sauce may also be prepared by hand on a board, preferably using a mezzaluna.

1 large bunch flat-leaf parsley

1 bunch fresh basil

a handful of fresh mint leaves

3 garlic cloves, peeled

100 g (4 oz) salted capers

100 g (4 oz) salted anchovies

2 tablespoons red wine vinegar

5 tablespoons extra virgin olive oil

1 tablespoon Dijon mustard

Maldon Salt and freshly ground black pepper

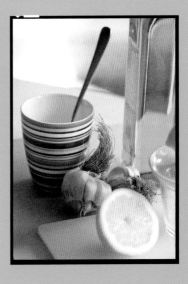

What's In *My* Larder

OK, so if Lloyd Grossman came round and did a *Through the Keyhole* on my larder and my fridge, here's what else he'd find...

✱ Fabulous extra virgin olive oil. I buy mine from The River Café and, yes, it's expensive: I am Mrs La-di-Dah when it comes to olive oil. But when I put fat into my body, I want it to be the very best quality that there is. Again, good fats chase out bad: many processed foods are still packed with hydrogenated fat, which has been linked to heart disease — whereas olive oil is packed with what are called polyphenols, and they are beneficial antioxidants.

✱ I'm not big on fruit. Fruit actually has a lot of sugar in it, and that triggers a bit of a rollercoaster effect. So I avoid bananas — which don't agree with my digestion — and I find oranges too acidic. I do, though, love berries: blueberries, raspberries, strawberries, blackberries — you'll always find them in my fridge because if I'm peckish, a little plate of berries satisfies my urge for something sweet. Berries are an antioxidant powerhouse, too, so I like the idea that I'm also helping my skin.

✱ If I haven't been well, I make sure I have yoghurt because that seems to help get my body back in balance. I buy the two per cent-fat variety, and it's delicious on top of those berries. But I have to be careful with dairy. I know it doesn't agree with me; it can give me the sniffles and it's not great for my voice. Of course, this is the same person who used to make herself bowls of custard when she got home from school — and who's been known, once upon a time, to sit down with a tub of ice cream and eat until I just couldn't face another spoonful. But once I *realised* that my body didn't respond well to diary, it made it so much easier to give up. (If you think there are some foods that disagree with you to some extent — but you're not sure — try keeping a food diary, and writing down what you eat and how it makes you feel immediately after eating and over the next few hours, or the next day. It makes it so much easier to work out what triggers bloating, or a breakout of spots, or a runny nose. Many health shops offer food-allergy testing such as various branches of Neal's Yard Remedies and Holland & Barrett.)

✳ Every time I make a salad or a soup I chop up loads — and I mean loads — of fresh herbs, such as coriander, chives, parsley and tarragon. I take a big handful and put it on top of the salad, or sprinkle it over soup. It's a great way to get a herbal health boost.

✳ I love wine — but the rule is that I *never* drink before I'm performing, because I honestly don't think I could sing with alcohol in my body. I like a glass of *good* red wine. If I'm sitting at home on my own, watching TV, I might have a glass of red wine with my dinner. I'm definitely not a wine connoisseur but my inner girly likes it if I'm out with a guy and he knows his way around a wine list. That's very sexy in a man. And on holiday? Give me a nice chilled rosé, when that sun's beating down... A friend of mine who really knows how to live introduced me to Laurent Perrier pink Champagne, and it helped me to realise that when it comes to wine, quality is better than quantity.

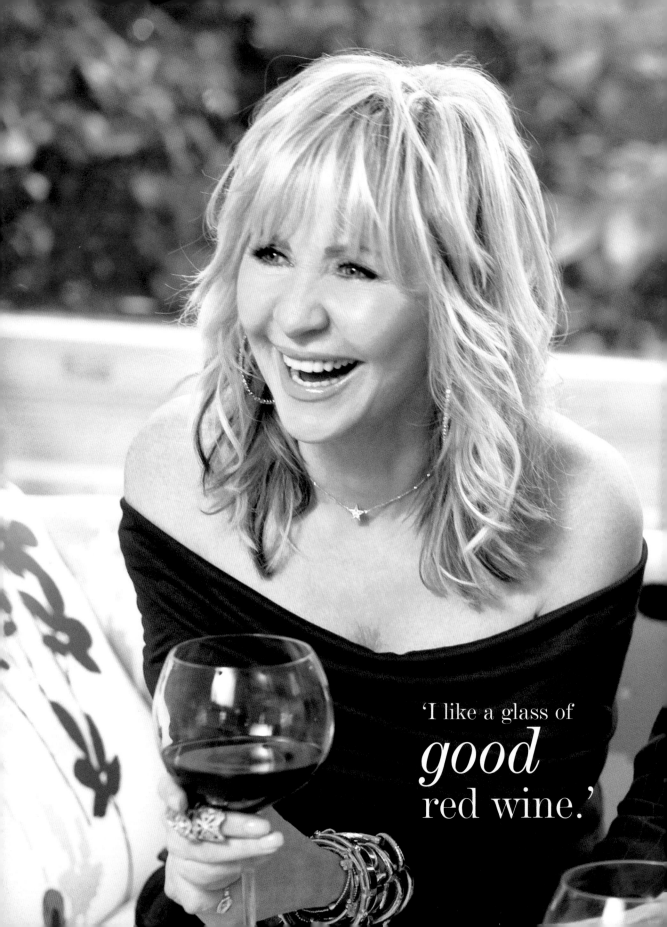

'I like a glass of *good* red wine.'

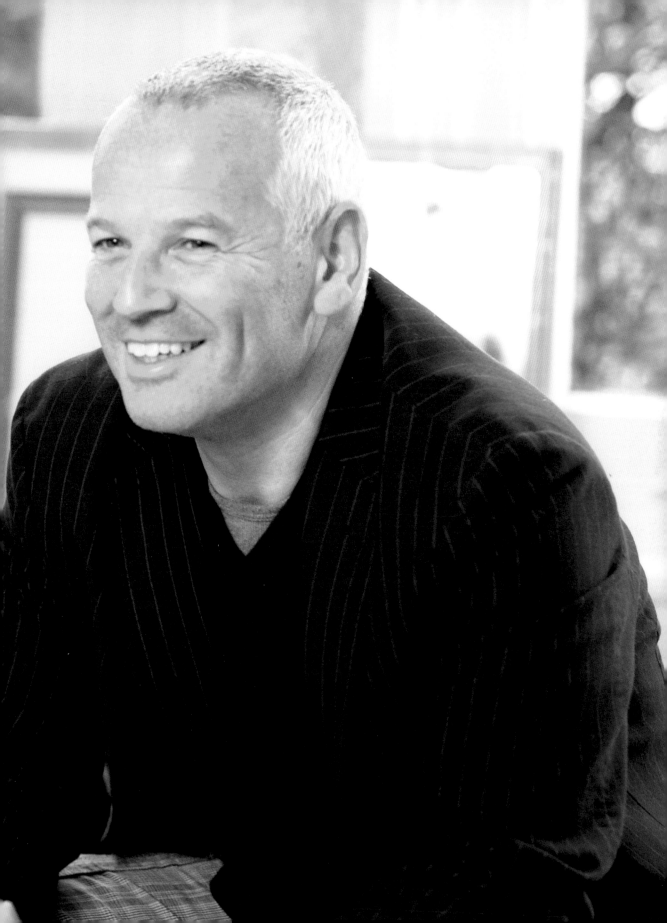

Sin-Free Brownie

Brownies are generally very naughty indeed. But this is sugar free, and really hits the spot when you have to have something sweet.

Mix all the dry ingredients together.

Beat together butter and cream cheese or mascarpone (both at room temperature). Then beat in the eggs and vanilla. To this, slowly mix in the dry ingredients. Stir in the nuts and then transfer mixture to a baking tin, spreading evenly. Bake at 180°C for twenty-five minutes.

6 scoops chocolate flavour Vianesse Professional Body Shape Protein Powder (see p.266) — use the scoop you get in the tub of powder)

7 scoops Xylitol (see p.267) or agave syrup

4 scoops organic cocoa powder

3 scoops Pysllium husk powder (Holland and Barrett) or Vitol Egg Protein Powder

2 teaspoons baking powder (optional)

200 g organic unsalted butter

200 g organic cream cheese or mascarpone

2 large eggs

2 teaspoons vanilla extract

1 cup chopped organic walnuts

My *Stay-Slim* Secrets

* I always keep plenty of bottled (or filtered) water in bottles at room temperature — not cold, because I don't like it chilled. I have trained myself to drink water; it's not the most delicious thing in the world, but I know it's good for me, so I make myself drink it. It helps keep me filled up between meals, but I don't drink it with food.

* On holiday I let myself off the hook completely. That's not to say I pig out, but I do let my hair down a little — no matter how good my intentions are when I leave home. I was in Greece on vacation not long ago and I ate a LOT of Greek salads, and I certainly didn't tell the waiters to hold the feta cheese! And in France, where I stay with Elton and David, the food is so fabulous that I definitely have three meals a day. But the key is to realise that it's a holiday from your real life, and from normality — that's what a holiday should be! But then you just pick up where you left off when you get home. If you've put on a little weight, it'll come off again once you're back to normal, so long as you don't try and starve yourself. Then you're back on the rollercoaster and, before you know it, it's all about chocolate and biscuits...

* I like a curry as much as the next person — no, maybe more! But I've eaten a lot of Indian food in India, when I've been on meditation retreats, and I've learned that it's very different to the food you'll find in most Indian restaurants in the UK, which is very high in fat (usually hydrogenated), and often straight from the freezer to the microwave. I have an Indian friend in London and she has helped me seek out the kind of Indian restaurant where they use fresh ingredients, fresh spices and cook from scratch. There is a world of difference: 'fresh' Indian food is very clean, not a glutinous sloppy mess. When I eat curry, though, I tend to go for chapatis, plain naans and popadums. I used to be terribly brown-rice-and-Woodstock in the 1960s, but I'm not big on rice now.

* If I've been overindulging, I know now that it's likely to be because I'm stressed, travelling or not getting enough sleep. My clothes tell me soon enough — and it's less stressful to find out that you've put on a few pounds from a waistband being a bit tight than staring at figures on a scale. (Besides, women's weight naturally fluctuates by a few pounds over the course of a month, so the scales don't tell you much. I gave up mine years ago.) It's hard to eat regular meals when I'm touring — and pretty fatal when I've been touring with Jools Holland, because he LOVES his food! But I do the best I can. I try to stay positive by reminding myself that when the tour is over, I can get back to normal and get back into good habits.

'I LIKE A CURRY AS MUCH AS THE NEXT PERSON – NO, MAYBE MORE!'

✳ I try not to eat pasta often. Like most carbohydrate foods, I've found that it makes me feel sluggish and isn't great for my blood sugar. But again, I never say never. If I'm going out with my sister for a special occasion lunch — like my birthday — then a big bowl of steaming pasta is a huge comfort-food treat. But I've trained myself to like vegetables and protein, because I know that's what my body really responds to best.

✳ In the same way, I try to pass up the bread basket. If I have a little mid-afternoon snack before going out to dinner — maybe a slice of chicken with some mustard or salsa on top — then I find it's so much easier to 'Just Say No' because I'm not ravenous when the bread comes around. Because, if I'm really hungry and the first course takes ages, I'm going to want to fill up on bread.

✳ The rule: one dessert, lots of spoons! You don't need dessert after a meal. But you do usually crave a teeny little sweet palate-cleansing something... So, order one between you, and share!

✳ It was all about milk chocolate when I was a kid, but now it's all about dark chocolate — and it has to be Green & Black's. When you crave chocolate go for the dark stuff as I've read that it is packed with antioxidants — who knew? — so I can tell myself that it's doing me good, and just a square or two is satisfying because it gives you a great big cocoa 'hit' without all the fat and sugar. Having said that, I don't generally keep it in the house, because if I do, I swear it calls my name from behind the larder door.

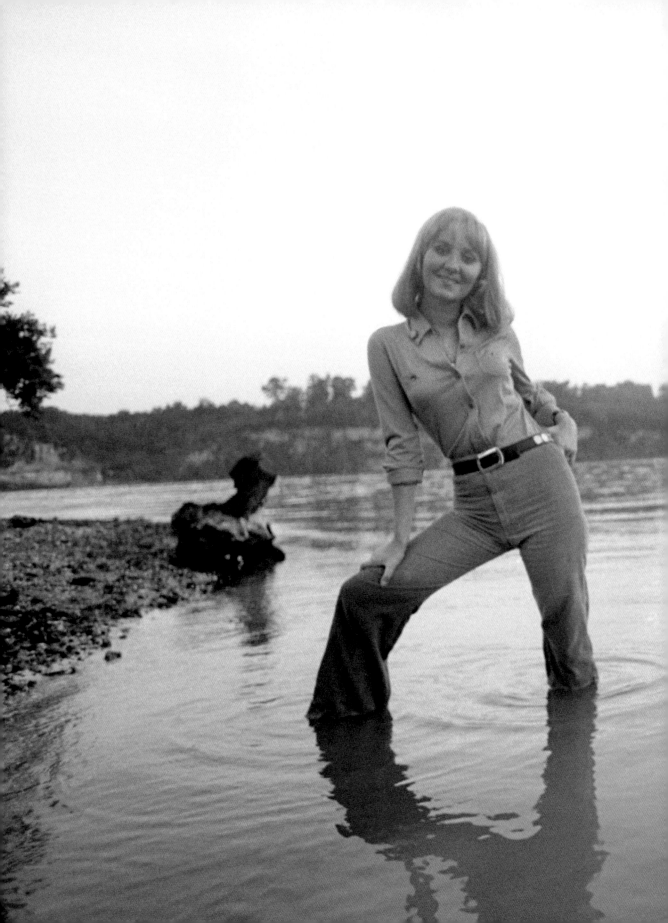

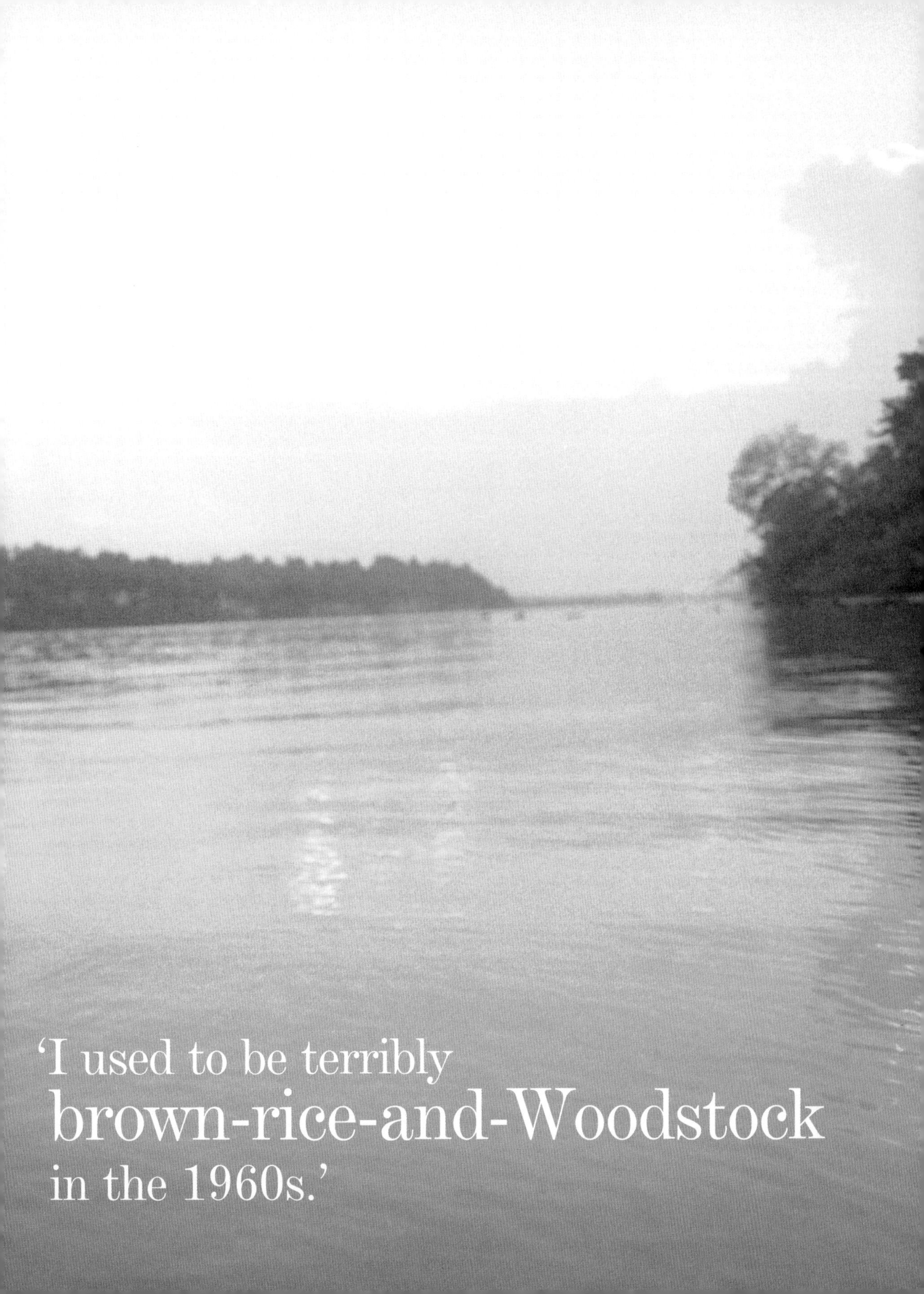

'I used to be terribly
brown-rice-and-Woodstock
in the 1960s.'

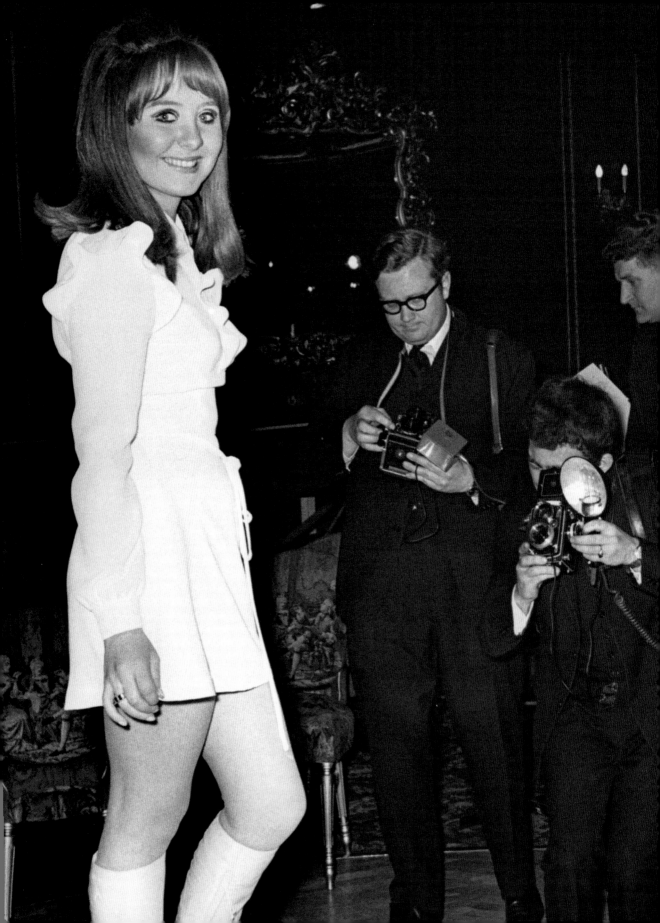

The Wardrobe Rules

Dressing up

I l-o-v-e clothes. Love them! Dresses, jackets, leggings, skirts, tops, cardies, shoes (oooooh, s-h-o-e-s...). And yes, I break a lot of rules because, in the past you got to 40 and wore neat little coats and cardies, and abandoned fashion to the younger generation. Well, not any more!

Having said that, I think every woman of a certain age has to have what's called a 'mutton-o-meter' built into their consciousness. That means not wearing clothes that really should be left to the younger generation (like my nieces), but picking out certain elements that do show you haven't lost the fashion plot, and still have that finger on the pulse, and can bring you right up to date and make you look fresh.

It's funny, but when I look back to the time before I left Glasgow, I dressed 'older' and more like a middle-aged woman than I do now. I actually used to wear some of my mother's clothes, and together we'd go to Wallis. Then when I came to London, I became tuned into fashion because my manager Marion's husband was in the rag trade — and, suddenly, designers like Mary Quant and Thea Porter, and stores like Granny Takes a Trip and Biba, were on my radar. I went to Paris and I remember the first 'designer' look I bought for myself was a pale blue-and-white striped sailor's T-shirt with three-quarter-

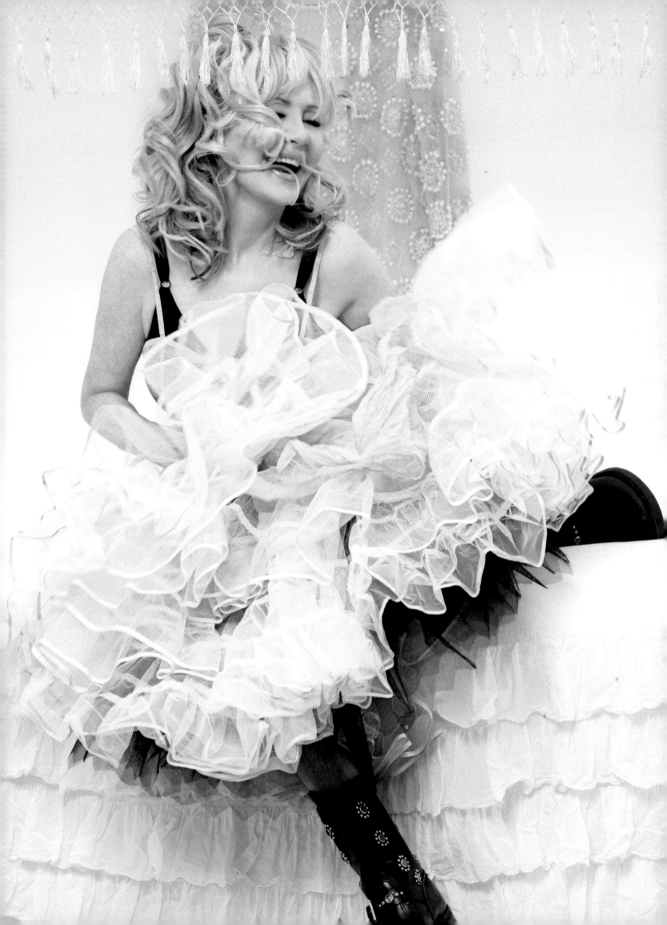

length sleeves, some denim trousers and some little flat ballerina shoes. It would have been a great look if the hair hadn't ruined it! Definitely ruined the Audrey Hepburn image that I was almost certainly going for...

But I was hooked! I still think it's important to know what's out there on Planet Fashion, so I read magazines, and I go shopping with my teenage nieces, to get my eye in at places like Topshop, Zara and H&M. The clothes may not be right for you, but have a look around at the women and girls in there: are they tying their scarves in a particular way that you could try, or are there some fabulous accessories that would work for you? Bags and jewellery in those chain stores are especially good as a cheap and quick way to update your wardrobe.

Now, you have to be a wee bit careful about this, if you've got a daughter, a granddaughter or a goddaughter to hit the stores with. My nieces are awfully sweet and they'll say, 'Auntie Lulu, you can get away with that. It looks so cute on you!' But I have to ask myself: is it over the top? Am I stepping over the line between fashion-conscious and, well, a wee bit tragic? Now, in my case, I have to be a little bit careful because I am short and can look quite girly in things. Yes, I like girly and feminine — but *cute*, at my age? That's not something I really want to hear nowadays.

But I do know I wouldn't give up my shopping expeditions with my nieces, and shopping with someone you trust — whether they're 16 or 60 — is really important...

Dressing well is all about proportion. I don't have a webcam so I can't tell what shape you are, but the key — oh, this sounds so simple, but so many women don't do it — is to play up your good points and play down your 'flaws'. (I don't like to think of them as flaws because I think every woman is beautiful. But there are bits of yourself that you probably like more than others, because you are *human*.) I am lucky in that I have fairly decent proportions: OK shoulders, my hips are quite slim, my legs aren't longer than my body (which is the one body change I'd like to make! Oh, for legs up to *here*.) But here's an example: I've learned to make my legs look much longer than they are. How? By wearing slim trousers that create the illusion of length, and wedges, heels and platforms (I'd probably wear stilts if I thought I could get away with it!). What you're aiming for is a look that is balanced, top and bottom. You don't want a top that drowns you because it comes down to your knees, or a jacket that stops too high up.

Your Best Bits

Now, this isn't rocket science, but you need to identify which are your best bits. If you really don't know, ask! We've all got something that we can play up, to great effect. If you've got a waist, then accentuate it — not necessarily with a belt, if that's going too far, but with clothes that have waists. (Actually, even if you haven't got a waist, I agree with my friend Susannah Constantine, who believes that clothes should fit the body's curves, even if you're a little bit on the larger side, because they give you a shape. Now, I love a kaftan or a 'hippy-dippy' top, too — but what you have to avoid is too much material so that it looks bulky; a loose-ish garment should still have a shape. Shapeless, tent-like garments will lead people to imagine that you're much bigger than you really are. (Hopefully, in this book, I've helped to infuse you with a little more body-confidence, a little more self-esteem — and, if you're less-than-happy with the shape you're in, maybe a few insights into what you can do to shape up, or slim down. But, meanwhile, don't hide yourself away under smocks and loose clothing!)

Find your
Fashion
Feet...

The Perfect Shape

Of course my shape has changed over the years — and, in some ways, for the better, thanks to yoga and all the walking that I do. When it was terribly fashionable in the 1960s to have a 'gap' between your thighs, I really didn't have one; you couldn't see a chink when I put my thighs together! But yoga and dancing have tightened my inner thighs, so that now, they're slightly concave and (which is THRILLING to anyone who lived through the 1960s), you can see a little daylight between them. So of *course* I'm going to accentuate that, because it's something I'm really happy about. I tend to do this with leggings or cigarette trousers (these are slim-line, fairly snug in the thigh and then straight beneath the knee). It's a look that the legendary designer Yves Saint Laurent perfected, and it is very flattering — particularly with a long-line jacket that stops at the thinnest bit... (I've found this is much more flattering than skinny jeans which cling around the ankle: tight around the ankle makes me look like Charlie Chaplin!) On the other hand, if your ankles are the part of your legs that you're happiest with, try a skirt that flares out and stops mid-calf, showcasing the ankle (a bit like Christian Dior's 'New Look' in the 1950s). Or a pair of capri trousers that stop just beneath the calf, showing off those slim ankles. The rule is this easy: identify your best bits and play them up. And *that's* what everyone will notice, every time.

I am quite small, so I have to be careful not to be overwhelmed by clothes and fashions. Much as I might love big, voluminous dresses, they are a total fashion faux pas for me. Because, it's a fact: if you're petite, you need to keep things pretty simple. (I have tried Princess Diana-style ruffles and they are absolutely not me — I don't look like Lulu, I look like someone in her big sister's dressing-up clothes.) So I like to stick to classics — with a bit of a twist — and add excitement and a fashion kick with accessories. Texture is important, too: I like to mix up fabrics: silk, velvet, cashmere, maybe a fake fur collar on a wool coat. It's a subtler way of adding interest than wearing lots of colours or prints, which can easily overwhelm.

If you're taller and more Amazonian, maybe you can afford to be a little more daring with prints, frills, etc, but personally I think it looks better to go for 'simple with a twist'. I do like my clothes to have a little bit of an edge, a little rock 'n' roll kick, which is easier to achieve with accessories than with actual garments. Look in my wardrobe and you'll see very few prints: mostly black, navy, some brightly coloured 'underneaths', accessories and basics, but only occasionally a brightly coloured jacket or coat. They're too memorable! All you'll hear is, 'Oh, I've *always* loved you in that bright fuchsia coat...' I have a couple of red jackets which I absolutely LOVED but they'll never see the light of day again because once I'd worn them out a few times, people remembered I'd worn them before and started to comment on the fact that they recognised them. Classic colours don't stick in people's minds as much.

Something I avoid — and I think every woman should avoid — are clothes that have too much fabric around the waist. It's a fact: even if we exercise and watch what we eat, our waists naturally thicken a bit after 40; the body does a sort of shift around. (I refuse to mention the words 'middle-aged spread'). We are not 'middle-aged'. We are in our prime, and it's not 'spread'!) So, if you keep everything quite smooth at the waist, that is way more flattering than lots of bunched-up fabric. You don't have to wear clothes skin-tight, but with fabric, as with so many other things at this point in our lives, less is more. Loads of fabric makes people think there's loads of *you* underneath, which is why something that fits a shade more closely to the body is way more flattering.

Be Your Own Stylist

Show a little skin. I really believe this: a flash of (well-moisturised) wrist or *décolletage*, an open-neck white shirt, a sleeve rolled up... You really don't want to be all covered up; I think that a V-neck or scoop-neck is much, much more feminine and flattering than being all covered up, because a neckline that dips a bit creates the illusion of a longer neck. (In the same way, although I like necklaces, I tend to wear long chains rather than wide, thick chokers, because chokers make anyone's neck look shorter (and surely there's nobody out there who feels her neck is too long!). If you feel 'exposed' in a V-neck or a scoop-neck, soften it with a scarf; but a glimpse of skin 'lifts' every look. Even if you've got a long, swan-like neck, a polo neck is hard to get away with — and so is a Mandarin collar. I know they just don't work for me (although I *will* let you wear a polo neck on a freezing cold day if you're walking the dog!).

I think that what every woman needs is a 'uniform' — a basic look that works. (I've always thought uniforms were sexy...!) Who has time to stand around in front of a mirror each morning, trying on outfits? Have a session every now and then when you do that — and then establish your uniform. Use accessories to add a jolt of colour. You'll also save yourself a small fortune, I promise.

It's true: I've had to push the boat out a bit, style-wise, because of what I do for a living. Nobody would expect me to come on stage wearing a twinset, would they? But I think twinsets were really for our mother's era. And we should be thankful to live at a time when, style-wise, anything goes...

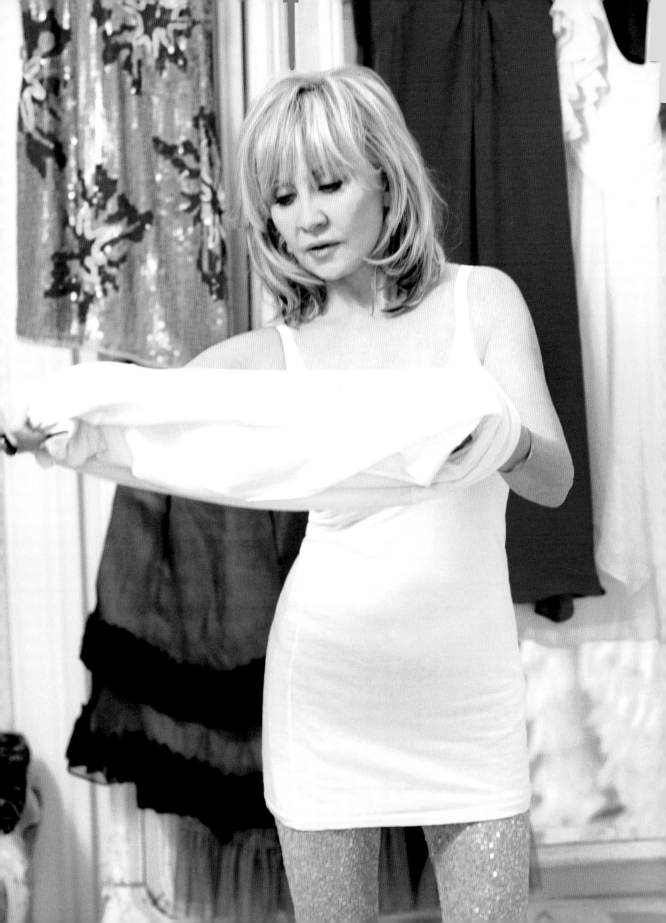

Baubles, Bangles *and* Beads

I have loads of accessories and jewellery — and a lot of it just comes from chains like Miss Selfridge (great for chunky, colourful bangles), Accessorize and Topshop. Jewellery is great for drawing attention and flattering your 'best bits': pretty hands, slim wrists, a swan-like neck. I like to collect bracelets: gold, Indian-style bangles and silver bracelets that I wear all jumbled up together on my wrists. (A great look with a jacket — try denim, or black velvet, with the sleeves pushed up.) A lot of them are stretchy, on elastic, so they fit snug to the wrist so it looks slender. (I picked most of mine up in America, or at Butler & Wilson, which is a treasure trove for jewellery lovers.)

I have colourful plastic accessories for summer to jazz up beachwear (now there's a word to strike fear into the hearts of most women!) and separates. My tip: rather than buying brightly coloured clothes, buy accessories in bright shades. They're a low-investment way of jazzing up your look, and they're much easier to pull off than a bright jacket or dress.

I spend lots of time people watching, and especially clothes watching. I am always analysing how someone's put their look together and borrowing elements for my own look. You can do the same, I promise, *so* easily: you just have to start looking. I went to the Brits with my record-producer friend Dallas Austin — he's an übercool African-American guy who has worked with Pink, Gwen Stefani, Madonna, and The Sugababes). Dallas was wearing a fabulous leather jacket with a cowboy-style bandana

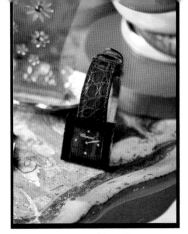

scarf and loads of chains with little buddhas or skulls hanging off them — and I just borrowed the look for myself. (I often look at guys and think I'd like to dress like them. If I go too unashamedly feminine, I get the 'cute' tag.) Now, maybe that's easier for me to get away with because I'm in the music business and am expected to dress up a bit (the skulls might not get the thumbs-up from your girlfriends, but I *love* them). But the truth is that you won't know whether or not something flatters you and zhooshes up your look until you give it a go. It's the way I am with hair and make-up, as I've said: I play and experiment and some of it works and some doesn't. But I know one thing that happens to women after 40, let alone 50 or 60, is they get stuck in a style rut. And that's not going to happen to me. Uh-uh.

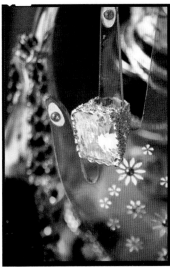

How you store your jewellery is really important: it has to be easily accessible so that you can see at a glance what you've got, and you have to make sure that it's not all jumbled up.

I hang up my chains — because if I didn't, they'd macramé themselves together and life's too short to spend it unravelling chains. When I travel, I take a sheet of tissue paper, lay the necklaces down lengthways and then fold the tissue paper along the length of the chain, then fold them in three. No more tangles! I keep my bangles on a kitchen-roll holder, and with earrings, I have some little Perspex dividers from IKEA or The Holding Company.

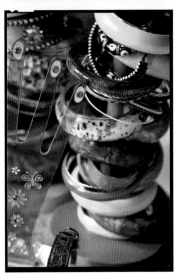

And I read another great tip not so long ago from Shirley Conran — mother of designer Jasper Conran, and the original 1970s 'Superwoman' — who keeps her earrings in ice cube trays in her drawers! One pair per 'ice cube'. Organising things like this is personal, so it's a case of whatever works for you. But if it's too hard to figure out what you've got because it's a giant mess, you're missing a trick (and a treat).

Kitchen-roll holders keep my bangles neatly stacked for easy access.

Sexy Scarves

I've probably got hundreds of scarves that I've collected over the years. Soft cotton ones, silk ones, chiffon ones... (chiffon is great for draping). I have a favourite skull scarf that I loop twice around my neck before I tie it. (There I go with my skull fetish again.) I have some fabulous leopard-print scarves that add instant 'pow' to an all-black outfit. Trust me: every woman needs some animal prints in her wardrobe, and if you feel that a leopard-print coat or a skirt is too daring, a scarf is a low-risk way to *p-u-r-r*, sexily, with what you're wearing. I also have some fab leopard-print plastic bangles. I slip them on with a plain black dress and some high heels and it's an instant party transformation. And I have an absolute rainbow of pashminas that I've collected over the years — some of them on trips to India, where they are amazing bargains. Pashminas waft in and out of fashion, but they're a perennial as far as I'm concerned; a really quick way to add a jolt of colour to a dark outfit so that you don't look like you're off to a funeral. Do you find that, at our age, it's hard to think of a present you'd really love? I don't think you can go wrong with slowly building up a pashmina collection

'PASHMINAS WAFT IN AND OUT OF FASHION, BUT THEY'RE A PERENNIAL AS FAR AS I'M CONCERNED'

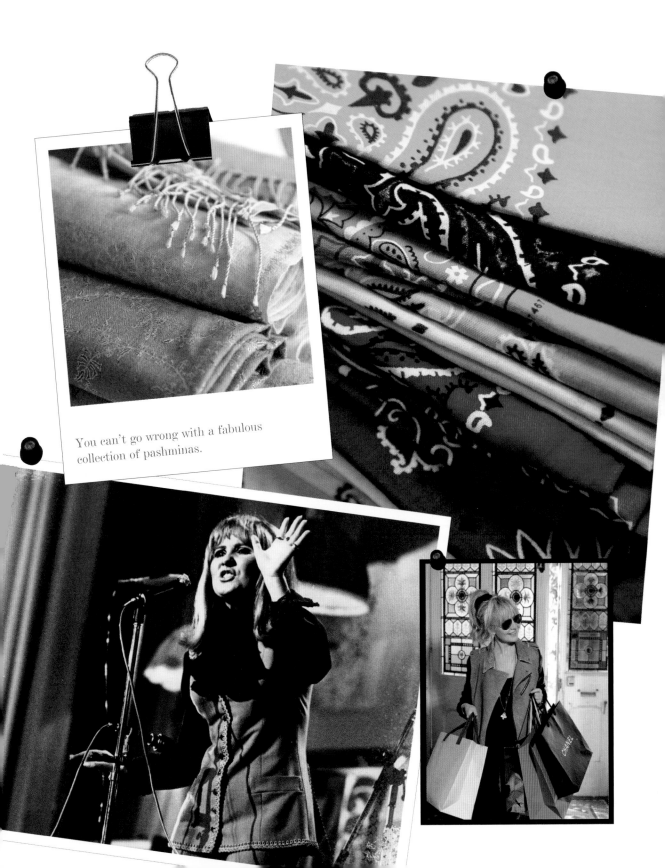

You can't go wrong with a fabulous collection of pashminas.

Going *Undercover*

Confession time: my boobs are actually bigger than I'd like them to be. I wouldn't want to be flat as a pancake, but I'm a 32 D cup, and that's tricky — because, frankly, almost all clothes are designed for women with no boobs at all. In fact, clothes are designed for clothes hangers — or women *shaped* like clothes hangers! That's why it's so important to try everything on. Nothing looks the same on the human body as it does on a hanger. A good sales assistant in a store knows how each garment actually looks on a woman — and it is absolutely worth listening to their advice and suggestions every time. They work with those clothes every single day — so when you find one, tap into her (or, very occasionally, his!) wisdom.

The most important items in your lingerie drawer are your bras, because they're so essential to help fight gravity, at this stage in our lives... Seventy per cent of women are wearing the wrong-sized bra right now — can you put your hand on your heart, or on your cross-your-heart bra, and say that figure doesn't include you? I go to Rigby & Peller (who also make the Queen's underwear!) for fittings, because their staff really knows how to measure and fit. Many larger department stores like Selfridges (and even some chain stores) now offer a free bra-fitting service — take advantage! I always go bra-shopping in a fairly fitted T-shirt with sleeves (and in a fine fabric) that hugs the bust area, because I want my bras to look good under that. That gives a bra the toughest challenge — and if a bra is fitted-T-shirt-perfect, then it'll look good under everything else.

You can use a bra to achieve the bust silhouette you want. I actually like my bust minimised, so I buy minimiser bras — and

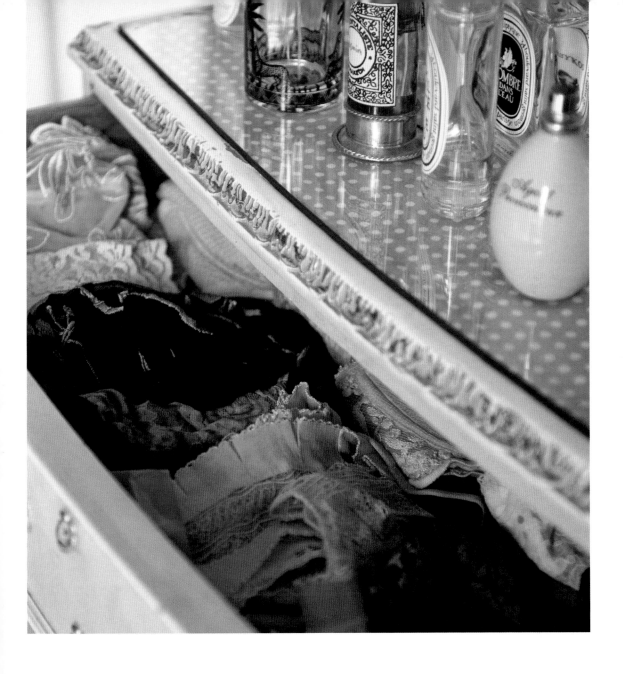

I don't want to hoist them up and put them on display. But if you've got it, *you* might want to flaunt it! Bras are amazing pieces of engineering — they can lift and separate, push out and flatten. You can downplay what you've got — or play up what you haven't. But it really is worth investing a little time — in a department store, or even a branch of Marks & Spencer with an armful of bras — to find out which work for you. (If you don't trust your judgement, take a friend who can be objective. And that T-shirt.)

For me, just knowing that I'm wearing pretty coloured underwear is an instant mood booster.

Pants!

I'm afraid I indulge myself here and wear a brand which is probably a little young for me — they're called Hanky Pankies. I've tried those big white Bridget Jones knickers and I just can't stand them; I like my flimsies pretty flimsy. Hanky Pankies are made of Lycra lace and you never have to worry about the dreaded Visible Panty Line — but they don't leave much to the imagination, either. I like them because they make me feel pretty and feminine, and because I tend to wear trousers most of the time so I don't have to worry about any lines showing. I first found them in the US — where they're made — but you can get them online here, too. I have them in turquoise, leopard-print, shocking pink and aubergine, black lace, black-and-white polka dots, plain white... Everyone should have a basic knicker 'wardrobe' of black, white and flesh-coloured — and, after that, you can be as daring as you like.

I sort of feel with underwear that it's whatever gets you through the night (and day). Like bras, knickers technology is really advanced now. Lycra means that you never have to endure baggy pants again — and with brands like Spanx, or Trinny and Susannah's Magic Knickers, you can buy lingerie that completely changes your shape. (A really good website to check out is www.themagicknickershop.co.uk.) The one thing you do have to be careful of is that, if you're going for a style that cinches in your hips or flattens your tummy, it doesn't all bulge out at the edges and give you a muffin top. When you find knickers and pants that you really love splash out a bit and stock your lingerie drawer. Manufacturers have a really unfortunate habit of changing the design once you've found your perfect pants and you can waste a lot of time looking for them again.

A *Different* Perspective

I analyse every performance that's captured on film and I look at what I was wearing, and whether it worked (as well as everything else about my appearance: make-up, hair — never mind the singing...). You can do the same, with pictures or videos that friends have taken. A lot of women I know don't like to see themselves on film, or in pictures. I say, 'get used to it', as it's a great way of reviewing your wardrobe and your look.

My very good friend Gail Federici, who worked with me on my Time Bomb skincare line, is someone whose advice I implicitly trust with clothes. Believe it or not, I'll sometimes get dressed, turn on the computer and show her what I'm wearing — from 3,000 miles away, with the help of a webcam! She might say, 'That looks great', or 'Uh-uh, put it back in the wardrobe.'

'A LOT OF WOMEN I KNOW DON'T LIKE TO SEE THEMSELVES ON FILM, OR IN PICTURES. I SAY "GET USED TO IT", AS IT'S A GREAT WAY OF REVIEWING YOUR WARDROBE AND YOUR LOOK.'

A Woman's *Right* to Shoes

Like almost every woman I know, I have a wee bit of a shoe fetish. Don't you? If I'm working or going out, it's heels every time — but for real life, rushing from A to B, you'll most likely find me in a pair of so-comfortable Converse All Stars (I have them in black, white, navy and a sort of beige-grey), which are great for dress-down days (and for travelling) — or maybe a pair of ballerina flats. (And at home I cocoon my feet in Ugg boots, which are the ultimate winter toe-warmers. I just think it looks sloppy if you wear them *out*, though. If you suffer from cold feet, buy your outdoor boots a half-size too big and wear socks underneath, instead.)

I have some beautiful evening shoes from brands like Manolo Blahnik. The reason you read his name in fashion magazines time and time again is because his shoes last virtually forever and almost never go out of style. Manolos are true investment dressing: a big outlay, but his clients wear their shoes season after season and, in some cases, decade after decade. (They're also perfectly balanced to make the heels *really* comfortable to walk in.) Christian Louboutin and Stella McCartney also make great heels — again, they're pricy, but a true wardrobe investment, provided you avoid the styles that will be out of fashion in five minutes.

Sexy high heels are a must in every woman's wardrobe. Somehow that extra height boost and strut gives confidence and suddenly you feel you can take on the world.

'UNSHINED SHOES ARE THE END OF CIVILISATION.'

Diana Vreeland

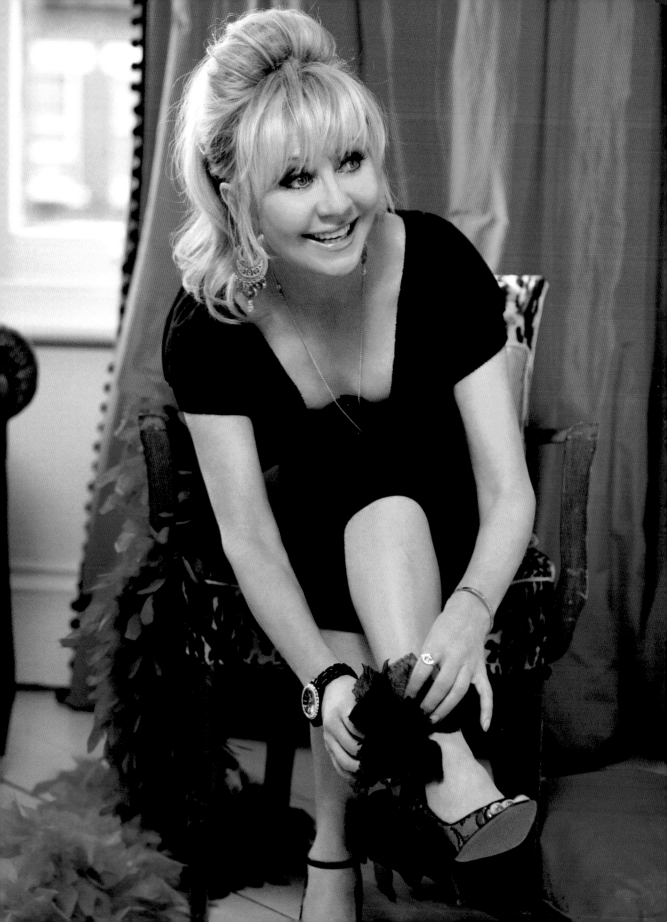

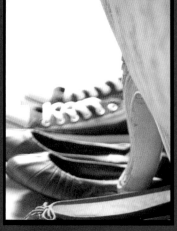

Shoe *Dos*...

✻ Practise walking in a new pair of high heels. Linda
Evangelista apparently used to tell young models to walk
around at home in high heels until they felt as comfortable
as slippers — and, certainly, that's a great idea with party
shoes because you do not want to get to the ball and find
out that your glass slippers (or, more likely, your strappy
sandals) are killing you. That pain will show on your face.
But if you wear your shoes in beforehand, that's a huge
help. If I buy a pair of shoes for performing in, I always
wear them at home first — but sometimes even that's not
enough and I have been known to kick them off while on
stage and sing barefoot!

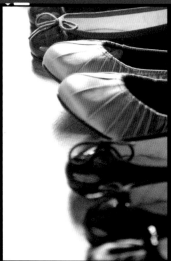

✻ Try wedges, as well as high heels. I'm a huge fan of
wedges, especially for the stage, because they give height
and stability.

✻ Take care of your shoes — you've paid good money for
them, and the more TLC you give them, the more you'll
get out of them. Buy shoetrees, get your heels and soles
replaced if they're wearing out, spritz them with water-
repellent and polish them.

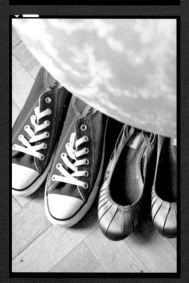

Shoe *Don'ts...*

✳ Don't wear a heel with a strap around the ankle — at least
not if you're wearing a skirt — unless you have Naomi
Campbell legs. In general, an ankle strap confuses the eye
and has the effect of making your legs look shorter (not
something I want to achieve!).

✳ Don't wear high heels with short skirts. Ever. End of story.
It's fine for your daughter (or granddaughter), but at our
age, it's a little tragic.

✳ You have to carefully choose the right clothes for
wearing flats. Again, it's all about proportions. I've come
to realise that flats tend to look best with casual jeans
or leggings and a long top.

✳ If you have an absolutely gorgeous pair of shoes that you
can't walk in — don't walk in them! Sit around at a party in
them. Wear them for a dinner where you know you won't
spend long on your feet. Enjoy them as decorative objects
and accept that, sometimes, women are just really, really
vain when it comes to shoes that are too gorgeous to
resist — and too agonising to wear.

If You *Dare* To Bare...
...*use fake tan*

Pasty white legs are very ageing with a summer dress — but who wants to wear tights when the sun's out? Even in my mum's day they used to fake a tan on their legs, using cold tea! Aren't we all lucky that cosmetic science has advanced a bit since those days? You absolutely *have* to tint your legs if you're wearing a skirt that stops at the knee, or with swimwear. For years I've been a fan of Guerlain Teint Doré, which is an instant (rather than a fake) tan which you massage into your skin and — hey, presto! — you look like you just got off the beach. (Ideal for those early days of summer when you throw off your opaque tights — and the sight of your legs gives you a bit of a shock!) Scott Barnes Body Bling is also *a-m-a-z-i-n-g* — very shimmery; it's used on photoshoots all the time when the make-up artist wants a really dewy, glowing bronze look. For more permanent results (which last a good three to four days), I've tried St Tropez — also good — but my new discovery is something called SUN, which I found on QVC. You use a glove to put it on but once it's there, it doesn't rub off — and the colour's fantastic.

The Long and *Short* of it

I think that you can absolutely get away with a shorter skirt at 40, 50 — even in your sixties. But it's all relative. We're talking just above the knee — and with the right tights. Black opaques make a short skirt possible — sheers are tricky to pull off — but black opaques are one of the greatest fashion inventions of all time, so far as I'm concerned. If you buy a good brand — like Wolsey — then you will literally have them for five years, maybe even longer, because the quality's so amazing. That upfront investment pays off because the 'cost per wear' — I love that idea! — goes down to almost zero after a few years. In summer, it's lovely to get a breeze on your legs — but obviously it's harder to pull off wearing a short skirt. I would never go for anything shorter than just grazing the knee, and I'd always make sure my legs were (fake) tanned, and that I wore flat sandals. Anything else just isn't age-appropriate, I'm afraid.

'I THINK YOU CAN ABSOLUTELY GET AWAY WITH A SHORTER SKIRT AT 40, 50 – EVEN IN YOUR SIXTIES.'

Belt Up!

There's a belt for every shape — even if you don't think your middle zone is your best feature. Very few of us these days look good with a cinched-in belt around the waist — leave those to 20-year-olds. But something a little looser? Or a belt that sits on the hips? If you've given up on belts, have a re-think. Go into a store. Try on some belts. Put them with trousers, or pull on a skirt and top and see what works — over a dress, under a jacket. It's my have-a-play philosophy! A new belt can *zhoosh* up an outfit you've had for years — and nice belts don't have to be expensive. I recently borrowed a great belt from my young friend Alex for a gig: I wore a black T-shirt dress, capri trousers and Alex's belt, which she got from a souk in Morocco — dead cheap, with lots of metal coins hanging off it. Fa-bu-lous! (And why not 'pool' some of your accessories with your best friends — so long as you keep track of who has what...)

'A NEW BELT CAN *ZHOOSH* UP AN OUTFIT YOU'VE HAD FOR YEARS.'

If you buy one accessory, make it a belt. They can transform any outfit in a second.

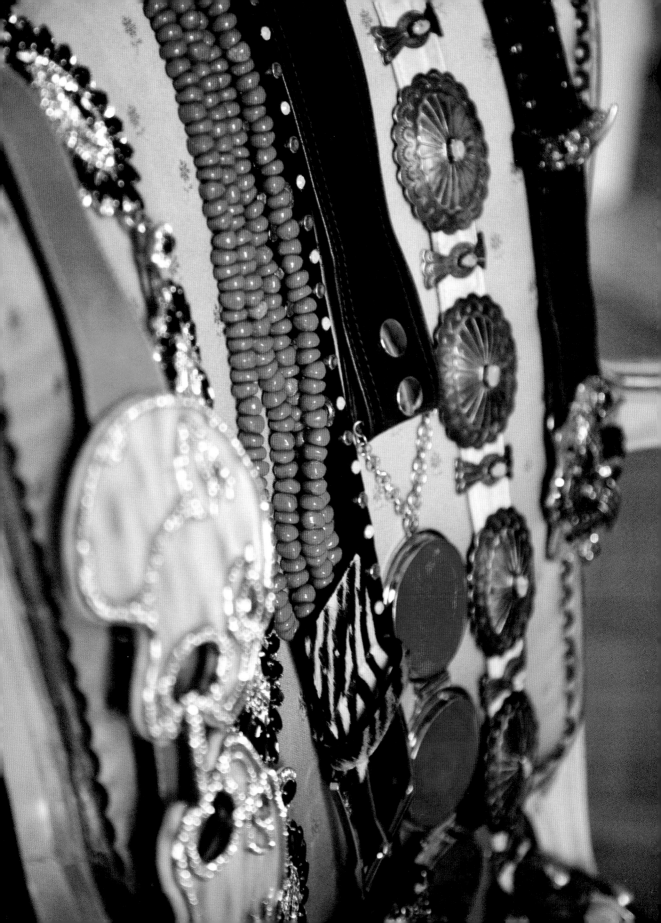

Lulu's *Golden* Wardrobe Rules

✳ You can't tell anything until you try it on. Don't just look at clothes on the rack, try them on — be brave!

✳ Find a good tailor, alterations person or dressmaker who can shorten, take in or let out clothes or change buttons for you if you're not nimble-fingered yourself. (Many dry-cleaners now have someone who'll fix clothes.)

✳ This opens up a world of fashion possibilities and you can also give your existing wardrobe a makeover with sexy new buttons, or by changing the fit of a jacket so it's less baggy and more flattering, for instance. A little tweak, a little tuck can make all the difference. Not so long ago I tried on a top that I fell in love with but it just didn't fit properly around the bust. My dressmaker fixed it — so much so that Simon Cowell asked me if I'd had my boobs done! It was a great disappointment to my mother that I never learned to sew — she always wanted a daughter who was a good dressmaker! But while I can pin things and even put up a decent hem, it's not going to stay put for long. So I've made a point of finding people who *are* good at that, and I get far more out of my clothes as a result.

✳ Identify a friend whose opinion you can absolutely trust and take them shopping with you, as your personal 'shopping advisor'. It's exciting! They can open your eyes to new possibilities, suggest clothes or combinations that you'd

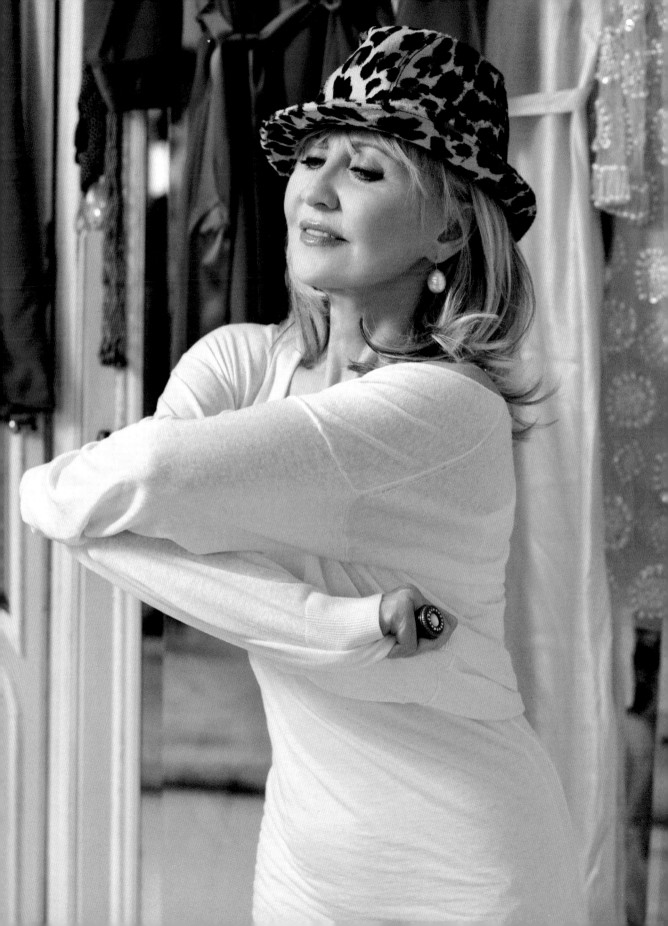

never have thought of and help you step out of a fashion rut. They don't have to be someone who dresses like you, but you should like the way they put themselves together. It's invaluable to have an objective eye.

✳ Go shopping with someone much younger, at least from time to time. It's a real eye-opener to try on things they suggest; you don't have to buy a thing — but keep an open mind!

✳ If a sales consultant tries to give advice, don't dismiss it as sales spiel. They're doing their job, and it's what they do day in, day out. Listen. Look in the mirror. Be open and be prepared to be surprised, because maybe they're taking you out of your clothes 'comfort zone' — but maybe you'll see a fabulous new 'you' in that mirror. I'll walk into a boutique or a department store — and if an assistant asks if she or he can help me, I won't brush them aside; I'll let them help, and be grateful for the insights.

✳ I play with clothes when I'm trying them on — I pull the sleeve down, or roll it up, tug at the shoulders to see how the shape looks when it's resting on my shoulders, or off-the-shoulder... I roll up the sleeves, I put the collar up to see the different effects I can get with the same garment. And I think it helps to have a bit of attitude with clothes — you wear the clothes; they shouldn't wear you! Don't expect to put something on and for it to be 'you' instantly — sometimes, you have to be a bit adventurous and *make* it yours.

✳ I really like a tip I once heard from Diana Vreeland, who was a big fashion diva and magazine editor in the US. She always advised getting ready — clothes, accessories, shoes, bag — and then looking in the mirror and removing one item — either an accessory or a layer. It means you always look chic and understated.

✳ Take care of your clothes, even jeans. They really *are* an investment. Even if I'm dog-tired, I hang my clothes up, and I brush them and get buttons fixed and make sure they're dry-cleaned as soon as they need to be. I've made a science out of shopping for the right hangers for different types of clothes: trousers, for instance, are always hung from clips, so you avoid that crease at the knee that is almost inevitable if you fold them over a hanger.

✳ In winter, I'm a big fan of layering — vests under camisoles under jerseys... You really do stay warmer with lots of layers, and I don't think it matters one hoot if the hem of your vest sticks out from the hem of your jumper nowadays! If you have lots of layers, that's another way to ring in the changes. Slip on a different camisole, have it peeking out — maybe with a lace trim, contrasting colours or same colour — and it's a whole other look...

'YOU WEAR THE CLOTHES, THEY SHOULDN'T WEAR YOU.'

Now Stand Up
Straight!

The fastest way to lose five pounds and take off five years is to stand up straight. I can remember going shopping with my mum and I'd sort of shlump when I was trying on clothes — and she'd narrow her eyes at me and give me such a look! With boobs, the temptation is to hunch to make them disappear, but I've studied the Alexander Technique in the past, which really helps with posture (and so does yoga). As part of the Alexander Technique training, you imagine being gently pulled up by a string attached to the top of the head — where the *fontanelle* (the soft part of a baby's skull) is. You feel your neck lengthening. The arms should be relaxed and heavy, but not so heavy that they drag down your shoulders. Keep your back straight and your buttocks relaxed. (You don't want them to stick out like a duck's bum, or have a swayback.) In a relaxed way, put your shoulders back — even if you've got boobs and you're self-conscious about them — and open that chest. It not only looks better, it opens the throat and makes it easier to breathe properly.

I took up the Alexander Technique because I'd noticed on TV that my posture wasn't great, and also because I was getting a lot of sore throats. The technique was devised by someone who'd actually lost his voice, and it's fabulous for singers — Sting has been doing it for years — because it gives the voice more resonance. But, very importantly, it also helps you to feel more at ease in your body — and clothes sit better on a body and person that's comfortable in themselves.

THE ART OF WALKING...

I'm not suggesting that you really learn the 'model walk' — but I do think it's fascinating to watch a video of Naomi Campbell slinking down the catwalk, just for fun, to see how the pros do it. *Every* woman can master the art of walking with ease and grace. What you have to be wary of is tipping forwards. I also see people jogging, who put down toe first, then heel, toe, heel — and that's really tough on the hamstrings. Should be heel-toe, heel-toe, heel-toe — not clumpily, but *s-m-o-o-t-h-l-y.*

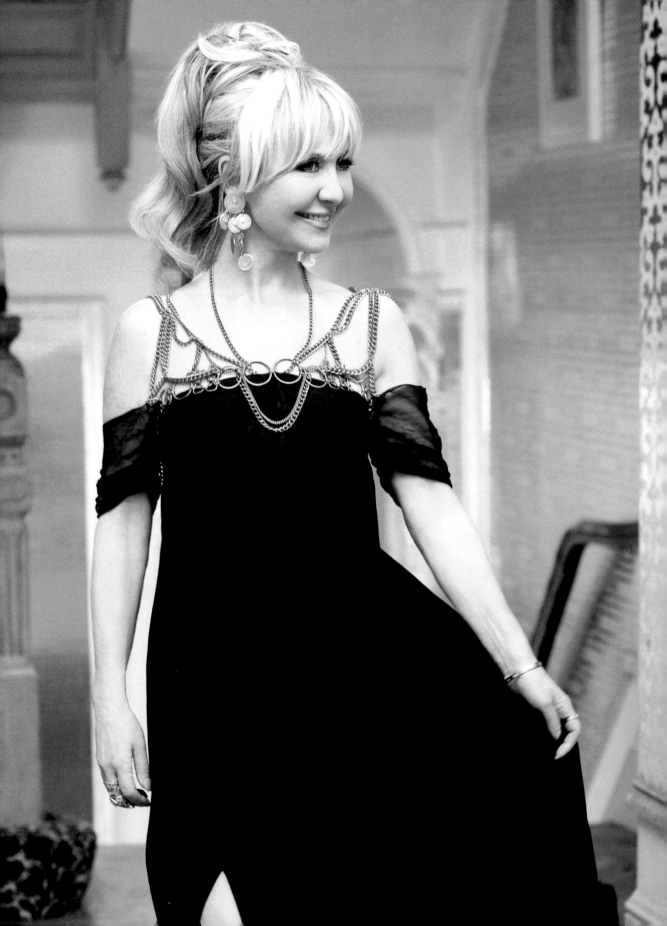

Must-Have Jackets and Coats for Every Wardrobe

A pea coat

This reefer-jacket shape is really flattering on everyone, and looks great with the collar up or down. Wear it with jeans, or a straight-to-the-knee skirt or trousers. Or try a duffel jacket.

A black or navy longer jacket

Nothing better! Can be double- or single-breasted, but if it's long-line — to just above the knee — then it can be worn with skinny jeans or cigarette trousers. My favourite jacket like this is almost teddy-boy in style with a contrasting collar.

Something stylish and toasty for walking in

Don't be tempted to sling on any old puffa jacket — look for something a bit more elegant, but which is really warm, so you'll feel like getting outside and getting your exercise. Ski shops can be a good source (doesn't matter at all if you've never skied!), because they offer far more stylish warm jackets than most outerwear departments. I absolutely LOVE my ZARA winter puffed jacket — I think it's one of my all-time favourite pieces of clothing — which has a hood. (I love hoods generally, because they keep my head warm.) It's down-filled and I can throw it in a suitcase when I travel and know it won't get crushed. (And actually, if I'm travelling, I can also bunch it up and use it as a comfy pillow.)

A really good winter coat

I think it's worth investing in quality here, because a good coat (the kind your mother would have approved of) will last for years. The January sales are fantastic for coat-shopping — you always find real deals on designer coats. Just be a little bit wary, though: there's a reason why nobody bought that turquoise trapeze coat when it was full price! Instead, opt for classic styles, preferably roomy enough to wear over a jacket without feeling like you're trussed up like a turkey, but not too loose and baggy. I always think that it's more flattering to have a coat that nips in at the waist even a little rather than hanging straight.

A well-cut denim jacket

Think you can't get away with denim? It's all in the cut. A tailored denim jacket can be worn with a pair of black or navy trousers and they'll look less formal. If you have a pretty summer frock, a denim jacket can look great over the top — but remember: it's got to have good shoulders and tuck in at the waist, so it's not too boxy. And there is a golden rule with denim jackets: it's jeans *or* the jacket — never both together.

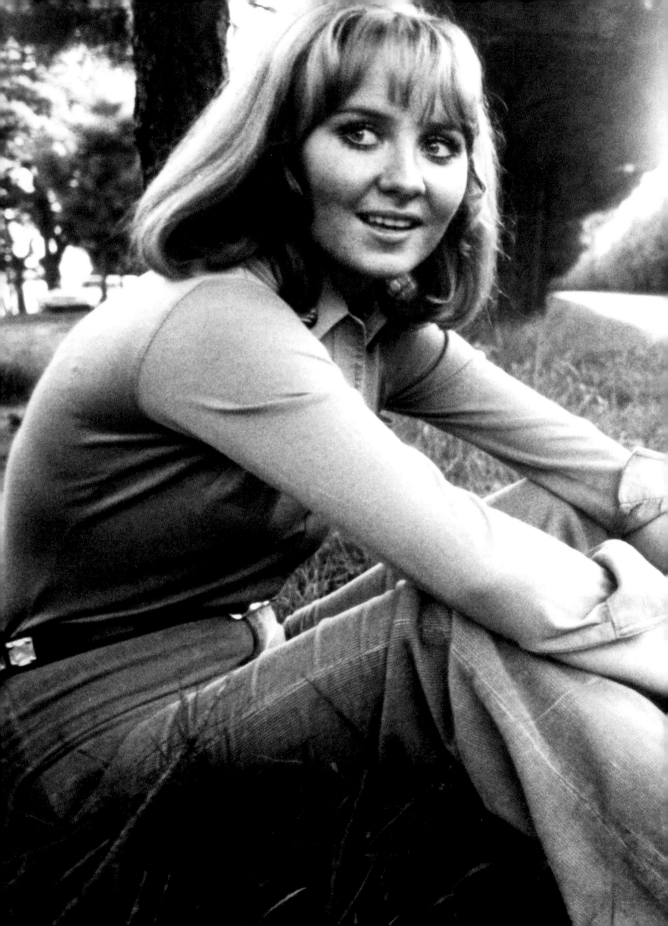

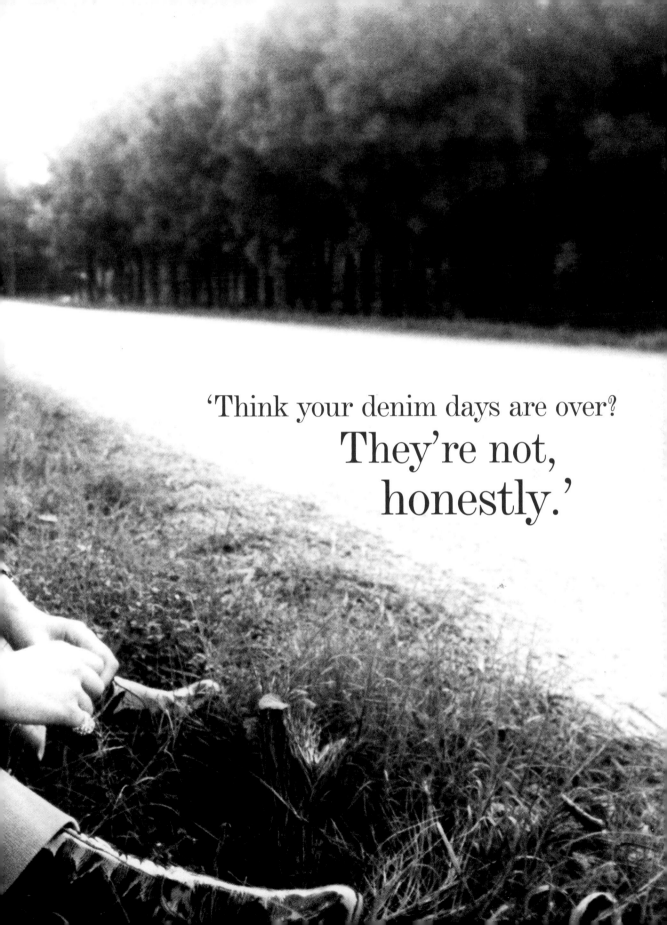

'Think your denim days are over?
They're not,
honestly.'

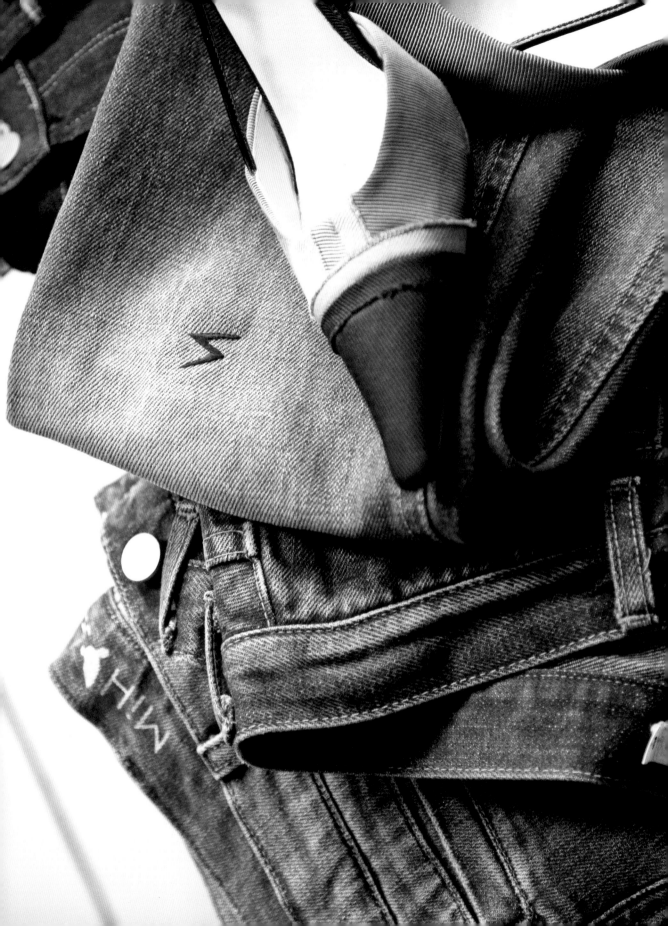

Pure *Jean-ius...*

Think your denim days are over? They're not, honestly. Even if you remember lying in the bath, shrinking your 501s to fit, or lying on the ground, trying to do up the zip of your soooooo-tight jeans in the 1970s, you've got to believe me when I say that, somewhere out there, there is a pair of denims for you. Obviously at *un certain age* you're not going to get away with the scruffy 'boyfriend' jean, with holes and faded bits. But tailored-looking jeans can be really flattering, and nowadays — you mean you hadn't heard? — there's Lycra in with a lot of denim, making jeans more comfortable than they've ever been. (A touch of Lycra helps jeans to keep their shape.) I've identified that narrow jeans and boot-cut/bell-bottom jeans work best for me — big, wide jeans look awful on me (because you can't see where my legs are under all that fabric. Wide-legged jeans are the equivalent of the baggy top: you want something with a little more cling. Not tight, but not loose either). The key with jeans is to make sure they fit well (but not too snug) in the waist — and, at our age, hipsters are probably a no-no. You want to be able to sit down in them — so do that in the shop. Make sure you don't spill over the sides of the waistband when you sit down. (And make sure you don't spill over the sides of the waistband when you're standing up in them, come to that! A 'muffin top' is to be avoided at all costs.)

I'm ashamed to say I've lost count of how many jeans I have in my wardrobe. My quest for the perfect pair of jeans is never-ending.

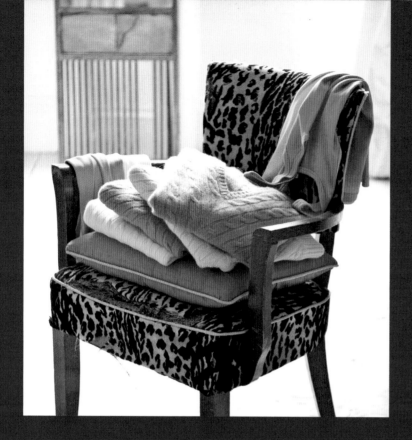

Very occasionally I'll wear something super-bright, but I always make sure that I team loud colours with more muted tones for a sleek look.

Just Add *Colour*

I think that the best looks take their colour cue not just from your own colouring, but also from where you live. For someone who lives in the country, all-black is just too 'city' (although black is perennially gorgeous, for every woman, after dark...). Rust, burgundies, moss greens — the colours of nature — have a place in your wardrobe when you live surrounded by nature. If you live by the sea, blue will magically look just right — from denim to baby blue via navy. For me, all black is a very metropolitan, almost 'London' look, and I feel comfortable wearing a lot of black, because somehow it goes with the pavements and the roads. (Black is also wonderfully slimming — and great on blondes.) White is another key colour for me, because it bounces light onto the face — which is always flattering. Stock up on white camisoles and 'underneaths' and wear them beneath a darker V-neck top or a dark jacket — then look in the mirror. It's almost as if someone switched on a torch.

My 'everyday' basic colours are black, navy, white — and then an added touch of red, brown, cream or orange. I'm lucky; with my pale skin and green eyes, I can get away with almost every colour. (I can even wear yellow, if it's just a flash.) Again — as with absolutely everything in my life — I like to play with colour and create combinations that work. (I have dressing-up sessions in front of my full-length mirror. Why don't you do the same? As I suggested with shopping trips, get a girlfriend round if you don't trust your judgement — or a sister, or a daughter...)

But here's what I love for my own style...

✳ *Black, white and a splash of red*

✳ *Navy, white and a deep Beaujolais red*
Think of the colour of Eastern monks' robes...

✳ *Navy and black*
Try it , you'll be surprised!

✳ *Navy and chocolate brown*
Again, a truly fabulous combination.

✳ *Navy or black and 'sugared almond' colours*
I love shades like pale blue, mauve, pale pink — very fresh, very flattering. But I really do need to balance them with navy or black, because otherwise I'd have to put on more make-up than I'd like. In combination with those dark shades, though, it's gorgeous!

✳ *Navy, white and orange*
Orange is a wonderful colour and easy to wear as an accessory, but not as an item of clothing.

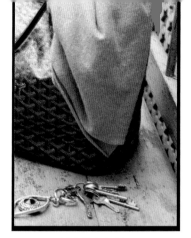

I am *Not* A Bag Lady...

I have gone off bags. Really, truly. I think the whole 'designer bag' thing was an aberration — I don't believe anyone should be under pressure to have the latest this, or the latest that, let *alone* something that's meant to cost hundreds of pounds and will be out of fashion almost before you've got it home. I just carry a shopping tote with me, with my wallet inside — you can find great totes everywhere (although mine are from a French luggage-maker called Goyard, and another — an investment piece — from Fendi). The bottom line is that they will never date. Carrying one (low-key) bag also saves all the hassle of constantly switching your stuff from one bag to another — file under 'life's too short...' For evenings, I have a little Swarovski crystal clutch that's just big enough for my keys, a credit card and my lipstick.

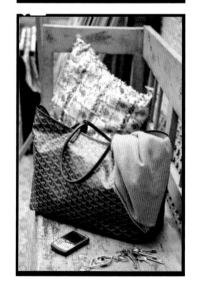

Fashion editors increasingly talk about 'vintage': it's 'green' (because it's a form of recycling) — but I think that when you are vintage, you have to be very careful about wearing vintage! If you wore it first time round, probably best to avoid it this time. I tend to look like a little old lady in vintage, and since that is the look that I spend my life trying to avoid, vintage is a no-no for me. The only good vintage purchases I've ever made are jewellery — an incredible Yves Saint Laurent necklace and bracelet, for jazzing up little black evening dresses.

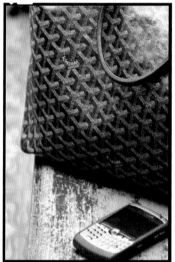

Let's Talk About *Sleeves?*

Why is it so hard to find clothes with sleeves? I recently read an interview with Helen Mirren in which she said she'd like to design a collection of clothes for more mature women — all with sleeves! I completely agree with her. As I get older, I go sleeveless less and less. Unless you've got fabulously, perfectly toned arms, it's probably time to give up on sleeveless dresses and tops. But you don't have to sweat in a jacket all the time. I've built a collection of shawls, pashminas and little 'shrugs' that I can throw over sleeveless dresses so I feel less exposed. Shirts over vests are good in summer — and if you're feeling really relaxed and confident about your body, you can slip off the shirt...

'WHY IS IT SO HARD TO FIND CLOTHES WITH SLEEVES?'

Dot Com Dressing

I used to love shopping; it was one of my favourite pastimes. But as I've got older, I can't be bothered to trail around the shops endlessly: I'd rather be having lunch with a girlfriend, or going for a walk in the park with my dogs. So now, I do my window-shopping in the comfort of my home, on the internet. There are some absolutely fantastic sites out there to help you get your eye in: all the catwalk shows, which you can click through to see what's of the moment. If I want to see the latest looks from Stella McCartney or Alexander McQueen, I log onto the internet and it's all there for me to zoom in on.

Now, I am not for one moment suggesting that you slavishly follow what you see there — no way! But in advance of the new season's clothes arriving in the shops, it can help you see

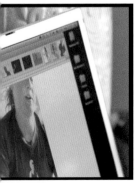
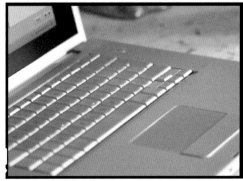
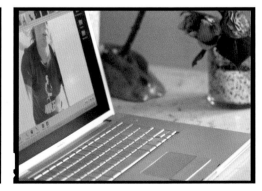

what's going to be on the rails in the upcoming season. Your eye adjusts. You can identify one or two key pieces, perhaps, that won't scare the horses and which would go well with what's already in your wardrobe, and then when you do go out shopping for something new, it's far easier to find what you're looking for. My favourite site is www.style.com, which has complete fashion collections online — and for anyone who's remotely interested in the fashion world, news from the 'virtual front row' is as good as being at a fashion show, but you can watch it in your pyjamas!

When I'm home in the evening, I also like to tune into fashion shows, sometimes, on cable TV. I especially like Fashion TV (and because I'm in the music business, I also watch MTV, to see what bands are wearing — but that's because it's my job). It's all about bringing fashion alive in front of your eyes — and it's an even better way than through glossy magazines, because you get the commentary, too. Sometimes I watch a show, and I'll run straight up to my wardrobe and try some combination of clothes that I already have, inspired by a look that I've seen on Fashion TV. I promise it'll do more for your style quotient than watching *EastEnders* or *Coronation Street*.

Browsing online is the easiest way for me to keep up-to-date with current trends and see what's hot and 'now' in the fashion world.

Some of My Favourite Things

I could cope with this capsule wardrobe — at a pinch...
(Although I hope I never have to!)

✳ A pair of ballet pumps — either black leather or black patent.

✳ Black jeans and navy blue jeans.

✳ Black leggings (or occasionally dark brown or navy but no strong colours) and narrow cigarette trousers.

✳ A black or navy blue soft jacket.

✳ Little cardigans — white, pink, cream and black, any colour, actually (they're a great way to introduce colour into your wardrobe). Long or short cardigans are all good...

✳ A pea coat.

✳ Shrugs — these are like little 'boleros' that you shrug onto your shoulders — love them!

✳ Some good quality T-shirts (you get what you pay for with T-shirts — cheap ones are ready for the bin after a couple of washes, if not before, whereas a good-quality T-shirt will last for years) — Gap, Velvet, Theory, JVL, James Perse, Rick Owens.

✳ Stretchy silver bracelets — from Butler & Wilson, Topshop, Miss Selfridge, and Browns, Loree Rodkin when I'm feeling more extravagant.

✳ Converse All Star trainers — the plimsoll-style, in lots of different colours.

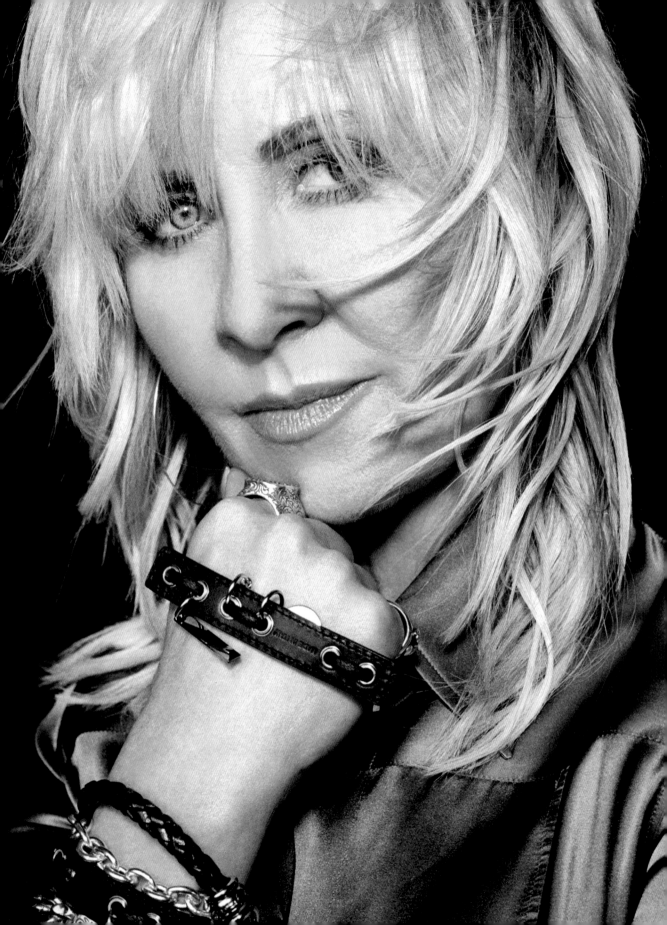

Mirror, Mirror, On The Wall

By now you will have realised that I analyse *everything* — but when it comes to clothes, a full-length mirror is absolutely crucial. I will stand in front of the mirror and look at myself from different angles to see how combinations of clothes look on me (a little hand mirror can help here, so you can see your rear view). It's nice if you can have a friend come round and do this together — it's always fun — or several friends! Women have this tendency to put ourselves down — 'Oh, my bum's so big' — but a girlfriend will say, 'Oh, but look at that gorgeous waist!' And maybe you should be playing up that gorgeous waist more with what you wear.

Still, there are mirrors, and there are *mirrors*. Some make you look far worse than in real life (and it defies belief that some shops actually have mirrors that make you look a stone heavier than you are. How do they sell *anything*?). Some mirrors, though, seem to make you look taller and slimmer than in real life. You know what? If that helps you to feel good about yourself, then get one of those. Take a look at yourself in that flattering mirror just before you go out the door, and that little confidence boost will make you stand a little taller, and smile. And that's what other people notice. Mirror, mirror, on the wall, who's the fairest of them all? Well, that's *you*...

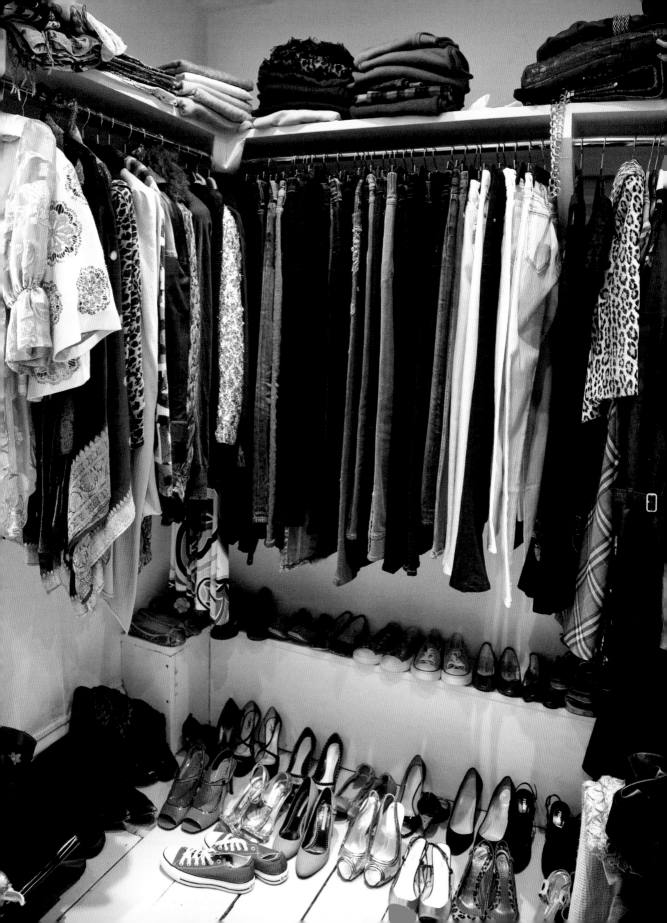

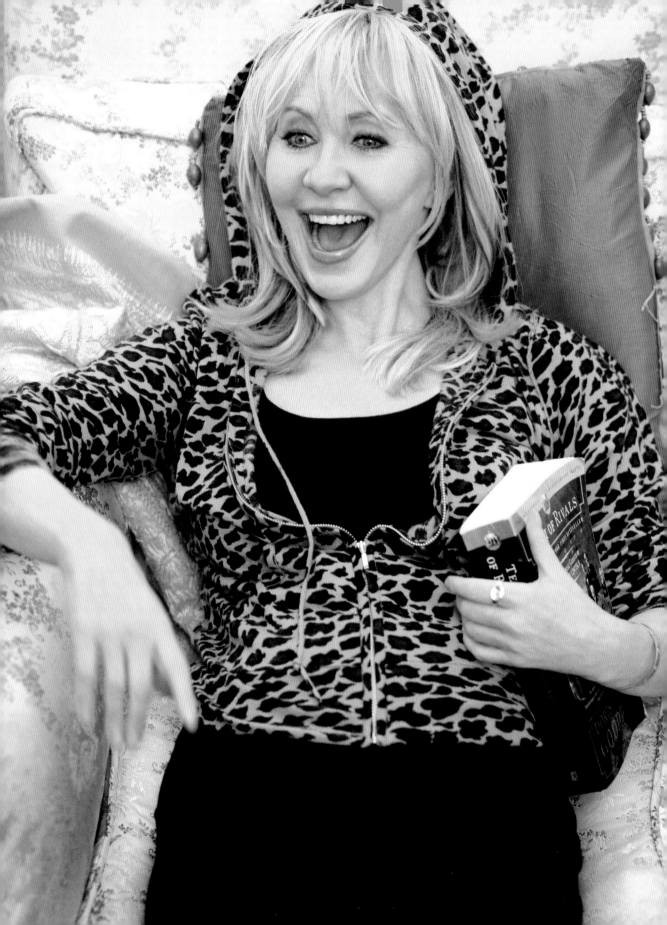

Beauty From Within

A Beautiful
Mind

Have you noticed how older people become stuck in their ways?
I am determined not to be like that. My mind is always open —
eager to learn, to improve myself. Having left school so early, I
am really self-taught in so many things — always seeking,
always looking for answers and enlightenment. I go to lectures.
I spend time in galleries looking at paintings and photographs,
to stimulate my senses. I want to go on learning and learning.
Not so long ago, I spent a whole day listening to four amazing
lectures by professors from America's Ivy League colleges, on
subjects like philosophy and economics, and it gave me a taste
to do an Open University course. If you want to stay as agile as
possible, that means keeping the mind agile, too.

'THE ULTIMATE LESSON ALL OF US HAVE
TO LEARN IS UNCONDITIONAL LOVE,
WHICH INCLUDES NOT ONLY OTHERS BUT
OURSELVES AS WELL.'

Elisabeth Kubler-Ross

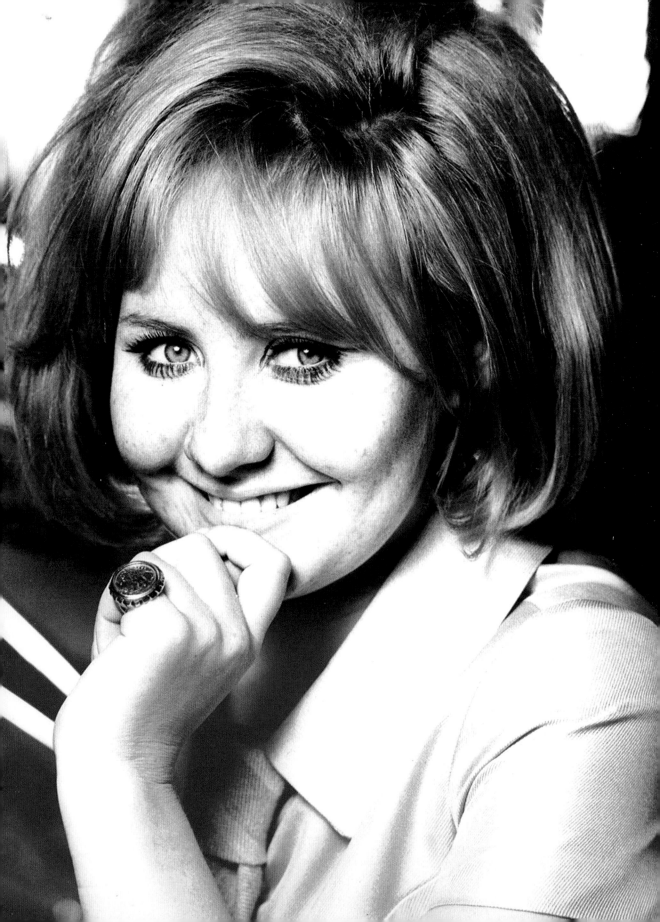

I believe that when you are engaged with the world in this way, it shines out from within — and makes you a more attractive person. We all know people who are resistant to change and have closed minds — is that attractive? No, I don't think so either. As children, we are learning and watching and drinking in the world, almost like human sponges. Why give that up as we get older? Step outside your comfort zone sometimes. Be spontaneous. Do things that excite you and make you feel alive. For me, that's all part of nurturing beauty from within.

Officially, I left school at 15, but it was 14, really — I couldn't wait to get out. I was ready, in a rush; I felt grown-up enough and I just wanted to explore the world that I knew was out there. At that stage, education didn't matter to me. But there really is a 'University of Life', and I enrolled in that instead. I absolutely do not regret missing out on a more formal education: my life has been like a Cinderella story, and that's my journey. But I had to educate myself, and I go on educating myself. In the past, I was often too shy to ask questions — although I'd drink everything in. What I've learned now is that it pays to ask questions. I remember early on in my career being taken to the White Elephant restaurant, and someone ordered *escargots*, and I said I'd have them as well. And, of course, they turned out to be snails! I ate them — I figured I'd eaten whelks, so what was the difference —but I was still in a state of shock, and it taught me not to be too shy to ask. If someone uses a word I'm not familiar with, I get out my big Oxford English Dictionary and look it up. Sometimes I sit and *read* dictionaries because I find that they really stimulate my mind. And my sister Edwina and I subscribe to www.dictionary.com which sends you a new 'word of the day' to learn.

As you'll have learned by now, I am a big believer in accentuating the positive — it's what I'm all about. It's how I've made the best of my hair, my skin, my body; it's how a wee girl from Glasgow managed to get herself a career that has lasted for over four decades — and whoever would have thought I'd be writing a book about my health and beauty secrets at my age? But it just goes to show what's possible, with the right mindset.

I've spent a lot of time in America, where people are generally more positive and can-do, and I think that's my natural attitude to life. But just as important as what you do for yourself on the outside — all the time and money you spend seeking glowing skin, or shiny hair, or a stylish look — is time that's spent on the inner you. Maybe the results aren't as instant as having a facial or having your hair done. But by working, gently and slowly, on your self-esteem and your 'inner' beauty, you will become more radiant. I have often observed that very spiritual people have a sort of inner radiance and tranquillity which shines out. You might like to start here...

'THE INTELLECT HAS LITTLE TO DO ON THE ROAD TO DISCOVERY. THERE COMES A LEAP IN CONSCIOUSNESS, CALL IT INTUITION OR WHAT YOU WILL, AND THE SOLUTION COMES TO YOU AND YOU DON'T KNOW HOW OR WHY.'

Albert Einstein

Finding a *Happy* Place

What did you do today that was positive?

Maybe you were extra-kind to someone. Maybe someone paid you a lovely compliment. Perhaps you met a person for the first time who inspired you. Before you go to sleep, go over the positive things that happened to you that day. While we sleep, our mind 'files' memories for future reference. If our last thoughts before bedtime are positive, it should help for sweeter dreams — and waking up happier tomorrow.

Smile

My mum would say, 'It's nice to smile at people' — and she was right. It's a nice thing to do — think how *you* feel when someone smiles at you.

Don't just smile – laugh! Laugh!

If I can't bust my stress myself, I go and see a movie or a concert with friends — or just get together and have a laugh. Laughter takes you outside of yourself...

Rewind the tape when you catch yourself having negative thoughts

As well as accentuating the positive, eliminate the negative. This doesn't mean turning into Pollyanna — but it does mean stopping yourself from giving space in your head to negative thoughts about yourself, which can so easily creep in. Whenever you catch yourself mentally putting yourself down — telling yourself you've 'never been any good' at this, or 'can't

do' that — stop and pause. Take a breath. Rewind. And remind
yourself about something you are good at, or you can do...

Live in the moment

In a world in which there's way too much to do in too little time,
we don't spend enough of that time just being in the moment.
Take a breath. Be here now. Stop, look around you and listen.
(Whenever I hear birds chirping in the city, I remember
someone saying they're 'like little angels singing at you...') For
a precious moment or two, don't think about everything that's
on your To Do List, or where you've got to be, or the pile of
laundry that's calling your name: appreciate the view, the
sounds around you, the colours or the way the light's coming
through the window. Hurtling through life makes it go faster all
the time, so stop and enjoy the moment. It is the fastest way I
know to slow the pace of life down again.

Practice gratitude

I consciously practice being grateful for what I have, instead of
moaning about what I don't have. (Because I do do that!) It can
be helpful before bedtime just to review the day and focus on
what I feel grateful for.

Heighten your appreciation of beauty

Beauty isn't just about the freshness of youth, or the perfection
of supermodels. There's beauty in almost everything. By all
means surround yourself with objects that please your eye, get
out into nature and drink it in and develop your eye by going to
art exhibitions and galleries. But the Japanese have a concept
call *wabi sabi*, which is all about finding beauty in imperfection.
So look for the beauty in absolutely everything, not just in the
obvious places.

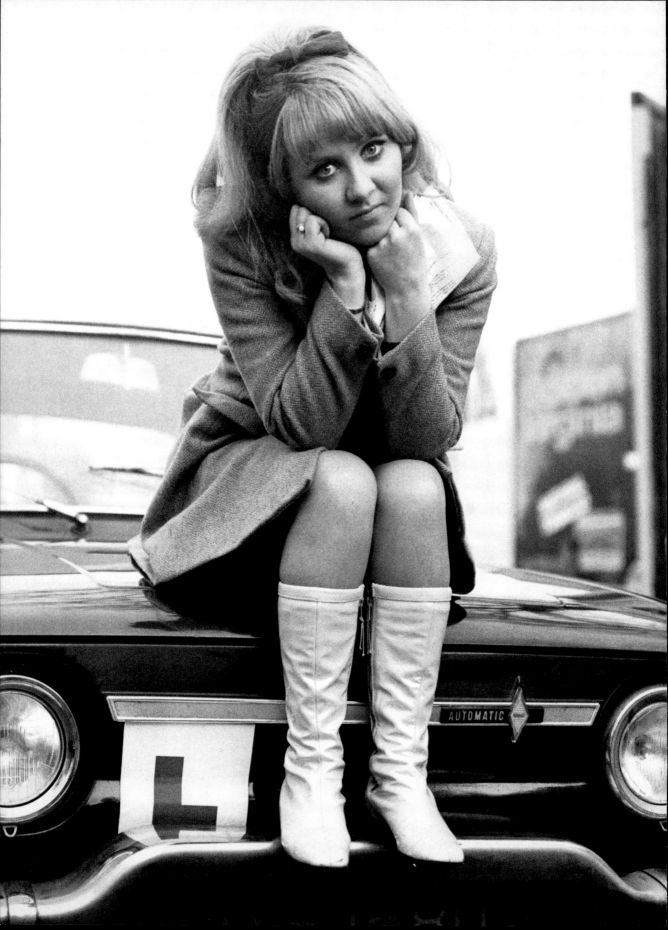

Be kind

Kindness is absolutely beautiful. Make time to listen to friends and love your family, but also be kind to strangers. There's a saying that many of our mothers used: 'Do as you would be done by' — which, in some Eastern philosophies is basically the same as *karma*, or the idea that whatever you do, however you act, this will be returned to you. I really believe this, and I try to be kind and polite because I hope that other people will be kind and polite to me. You can see kindness in people's eyes, and that is really gorgeous...

Be adventurous

Dare to challenge yourself! Once a month, at the very least, do something that's bold and daring and which other people wouldn't expect of you. That doesn't mean you've got to sign up for a parachute jump or learn to tightrope-walk if that's just not you, but join a group activity with strangers, or take a course in something you've always wanted to learn. Both my sister and a friend of mine have both joined a 'rock choir' — getting together with a group of people to sing rock songs. Staying interested in the world in this way is actually very good for inner beauty — and that 'engagement' is also intriguing and attractive to other people.

Be grateful

It's easy to focus on the 'if onlys', and what we don't have. Sometimes life can be very tough: we lose people we love, or jobs we love, or we don't get what we hoped for (although that's no reason to stop dreaming...). I like to review my life and be grateful for what I have — in particular the love of friends and family, and good health. In the same way that you review the good things that have happened to you each day, before bedtime check off the things you have to be grateful for. We should take nothing for granted in this world.

I was so disappointed when I failed my first driving test, but it was an early lesson in staying positive.

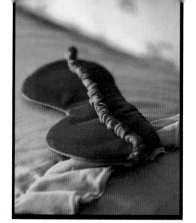

To Sleep, Perchance to *Dream*

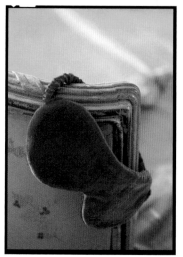

Sleep is the best possible beauty treatment — and it is absolutely free. The challenge is that, at a certain age — just when we need it more than ever, to repair our complexion (and our whole body, in fact) — it can become elusive. To be honest, I never get enough sleep. I am an eight-hour person — but I don't seem to be capable of going to sleep early; I'm a bit like a child resisting sleep... I am extremely envious of people — like a rugby player who I saw on TV a while ago — who can sleep for 13 or 14 hours on the trot. I get an average of six hours — but I'd love eight, and it does make a difference when I can actually manage that.

Most of us have got tricks that help us to get to sleep. A friend of mine actually has a programme on his iPhone that plays sleep-inducing music, and apparently when he listens to it, it's almost like being hypnotised — he's off to sleep in no time at all. To be honest, for me, it's as much about the 'don'ts', which include:

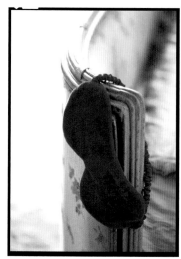

Don't write lists late at night
Fatal! I'm a real list-maker but I know if I do this in the evening, or just before bedtime, it gets my mind racing and I can't switch off. Different techniques work for different people though and if writing a list before bedtime helps to clear your mind, then go ahead and do it!

I often use eye masks on long-haul flights or when I'm finding it difficult to get to sleep, as they really do help to calm the mind and cut out the light.

Don't use technology late at night

No TV in the bedroom (no newspapers, either, because reading the headlines last thing at night is enough to stop anyone sleeping, frankly). So don't decide this is the perfect moment to sit and watch all the stuff that you've recorded on Sky+, because from a sleep point of view, it's not. So why don't you set a 'cut-off' time for TV in the evening — say 9 p.m. — and, after that, either read a novel or something very light, or meditate. (My son Jordan has also encouraged me not just to switch off the TV and my computer, but to do so at the mains. Leaving technology on standby still uses energy — and creates electro-magnetic waves which may not be so good for us, either. It's hard for me to switch off my iPhone and Blackberry at night — because I work a lot with people on the east and west coasts of America — but I try to be disciplined about it. Because of the speed of technology, we've developed this now-now-NOW mentality, but in reality, would it be the end of the world if something waited until tomorrow? It wasn't that long ago that we didn't have email, or even faxes, and did the world come to an end? No, it did not. But we've developed this sense of urgency which isn't good for our well-being — and definitely isn't good for our quality of sleep.

Don't exercise

I love exercise! I swear by it — but not in the evenings. If you go to the gym after you've finished work late, your heart and adrenaline will be pumping and it will make it much harder to slow down. Instead, create some kind of relaxation ritual. That might be a hot bath, or a shower, a hot (non-caffeinated) drink, a hot water bottle...

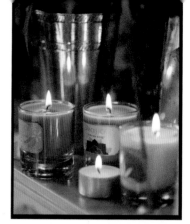

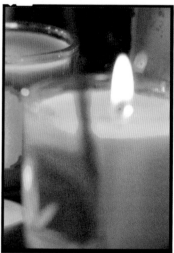

The Miracle of *Meditation*

Let me tell you, I have a cracker factory in my head. Given the chance, it's firing off here, there and everywhere with a million ideas, a million different thoughts and projects. What literally changed my life was learning to meditate. It helps me to close down the 'cracker factory' and get some respite — a reprieve from the increasingly fast pace of life.

You don't have to subscribe to an Eastern religion to do this or, in fact, any religion at all. It is simply an invaluable life skill, and something I do every single day of my life. It helps me so much to know that I can quieten everything down, shift my attitude, literally change my brainwave pattern so that I can access that inner stillness.

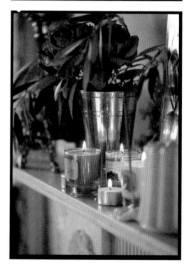

As with starting anything new, my way is always to find a great teacher. I don't kid myself that I can do everything without help. All cities and most towns will have a centre of some kind where you can study meditation. I found my teacher through a friend, who introduced me to *Siddha* meditation — and that's the type of meditation I still do today. So, my recommendation is to go to a class and have lessons. If that first teacher isn't right for you — if you don't feel a connection — then keep seeking. Eventually, the right meditation teacher will come into your life. This requires a little faith in the universe, but it really is the way it works.

People think that there's something mystical about meditation. But it's actually available to all of us. My teacher put it beautifully when she explained to me that, actually, we *all* meditate naturally: think of how utterly absorbed you become when you're focussing on a little baby, or a grandchild — you're completely absorbed. Well, meditation's like that, in *Siddha* meditation I was taught to turn that focus within. Personally, I get that sense when I'm singing. I feel absorbed, totally connected and present in the moment. So for me, because of my experience singing — when I am totally present, 'in the zone'— it is easy to understand what meditation can offer. (I love that phrase 'in the zone': it's the description Linford Christie used to describe his experience of running at the Olympics and finally winning a gold medal.)

I think it's really important to have the right teacher to show you what to do when you learn meditation. I'd been interested in meditation for years, but one day I found 'my' teacher — or did she find me? There's a saying, 'when the student is ready, the master appears,' — and, suddenly, I really understood what everyone was on about, and it was a revelation.

On a daily basis, when you start your meditation practice at home, there are some guidelines to follow. Have a space where you meditate that is peaceful, away from the doorbell and ringing telephones (and switch off that mobile). Do it when you're pretty sure you're not going to be interrupted — and, if you can manage it, sunrise and sunset are powerful times to meditate. Sunrise, before the world awakes, and sunset, when the world around you is beginning to slow down again. Comfortable clothes are important because you don't want to be aware of a too-tight waistband or trousers that are pulling when you sit cross-legged. Take your shoes off. I sit on a mat — and the more you sit on that mat, the more it becomes home to you. Then I light a candle. These are all parts of the ritual, and when you repeat them, day after day, the mind becomes almost programmed to become more still, even before you start to meditate. Trust me on this!

Practice Makes Perfect

Of course to do anything well requires practice — and that's certainly true of meditation. Just as singers have to practice their singing technique, in order to meditate, you have to practice meditating. And that really just means you *sit*. It's not about 'doing', it's about allowing yourself just to 'be'. To start with, your mind will fill with a million thoughts and you'll get the feeling you're never going to master this. Breathing in the right way is key, key, *key*! We hurtle through life and we even *hold* our breath a lot of the time, but in meditation, breathing really slows everything down. Take a really deep breath when you start, and breathe deeply and rhythmically, not just from high up in the chest, but in the abdomen. It can be helpful to learn *pranayama*, which is the breathing element of yoga (and most yoga classes teach a bit of *pranayama* along with the postures). In *pranayama* you count the in breaths and the out breaths, breathing though alternate nostrils (you press your thumb and ring finger onto the alternately 'closed' nostril) — and you hold the breath in before you breathe out again. Imagine a count of four as you breathe in, hold for four, breathe out to a count of four. That's the simplified version, but you get the idea.

'YOUR VISION WILL BECOME CLEAR ONLY WHEN YOU CAN LOOK INTO YOUR OWN HEART.'

Carl Jung

Like everything, meditation calls for discipline and perseverance. If you've found a good teacher, he or she may have given you a couple of chants, or *mantras*, to repeat. This helps with focus and with quieting the mind. Chanting is like singing; it opens the heart *chakra* (or centre), and the breathing helps to slow the heart down, and then the mind follows. After a while, you don't actively have to do anything. The ritual simply starts the process off and, before you know it, you're accessing that inner calm.

Do it Daily

Meditation can be done morning or night, and it really should be a daily thing. Once you start, it's really important to be disciplined, and ideally to do it at the same time every single day because the benefits are cumulative. I meditate for 20 minutes every single day. Sometimes, if I'm extremely fortunate, I will find time to visit a meditation centre near my house for a 45-minute deep relaxation. I have been doing it so long now I can even meditate in the car — although not, of course, if I'm driving! When I meditate, I get clarity, because meditation gets to the hub of the heart. Inside, we all know how we should behave in a situation, or changes we should make in our lives, but often, our head overrules our heart. Meditation helps to connect the head with the heart.

I have often had friends say to me, 'Oh, but I don't have the time to meditate'. In reality, though, taking these precious few minutes every day gives you an inner calm and an inner strength that makes it so much easier to deal with everything that life throws at you. And I find that it also magically silences the 'cracker factory'.

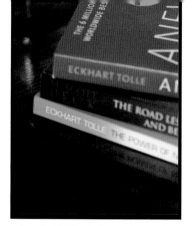

Health *Check*

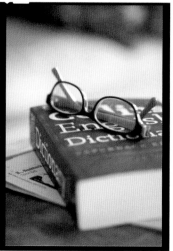

I do think it's important — a bit like a car — to go for a regular service: to get your health checked out, top-to-toe. When I hit 60, I had my 60-year service! I think it's far better to get a 'snapshot' of your health every 12 to 18 months — which can point to any early warning signs — than to wait for a wake-up call. Personally, I get that 'snapshot' — the usual women's tests, and a heart check, etc — and then I have a team of natural-health practitioners who I go to, armed with that information, to help me build up my immunity and rebalance me, if I'm at risk of running on empty. (Of course, if I had a serious problem, I'd head straight for a conventional doctor, but the idea is that, if you work at maintaining good health on an ongoing basis, well, as with most things, prevention is better than cure...)

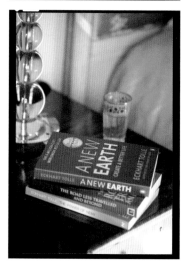

Over the years I have visited acupuncturists (acupuncture is fantastic for women who are menopausal), homeopaths and Ayurvedic meditation practitioners. What works for me might not work for you — and I know that at different times in my life, different therapies seem to have been effective for me, so it's an ongoing quest. But I do believe that we shouldn't wait until we're ill before seeking help, but should instead seek 'positive health' — building immunity and resilience to make us better able to resist disease. Why wait for something to go wrong?

The best place to start is with friends' recommendations — girlfriends can often point you in the direction of therapists who've helped them. If none of your friends take this approach to 'positive health' or have used complementary medicine to help with health niggles, then most towns have a natural health centre. And, if they're any good at all, they'll offer a free

I love to read, learn and absorb information, so you'll often find several books on the go next to my bed.

15-minute consultation with any of their experts so you can talk through your symptoms or what you're hoping to get out of a session, and also see how you feel with that person. (You want to feel absolutely confident in anyone into whose hands you're placing your health.)

I appreciate that complementary therapies can cost money — because you can wait forever to get an appointment for one of the handful available on the NHS — but it's a question of priorities. If you're feeling under par, which is more important: a new pair of shoes, or a boost to your health?

The expert I currently see is Dr Nonna Brenner — a doctor who's also a homeopath and a naturopath. I like to go to her Centre (which is in the Austrian mountains) for healing and regeneration. She diagnoses using a technique of Tibetan 'pulses' (in Tibetan medicine, we have several 'pulses' which relate to different organs in the body — not just a heart pulse). She creates a completely individual programme of internal cleansing, detox and homeopathic remedies and herbal infusions to boost the immune system, as well as massages based on vibration, to help regenerate and cleanse the organs.

'IF YOU'RE FEELING UNDER PAR, WHICH IS MORE IMPORTANT: A NEW PAIR OF SHOES, OR A BOOST TO YOUR HEALTH?'

I went to her Centre because my body had been sending out signs that I'd overdone it, ricocheting between LA and the East Coast of America and London, and I picked up a really bad chest infection while travelling. (Planes are terrible environments to be in: they dry out your airways, making you very vulnerable to all those bugs flying around in an enclosed space, and to fellow passengers, coughing and sneezing.) I'm used to having a lot of energy and pushing myself — and I basically still feel like a 15-year-old — but sometimes, the body gives a gentle reminder that actually, you're *not* a teenager any more. And at this age, recovery takes a little longer.

Sure enough, my visit to Nonna's clinic got me back on track. Now, Western medicine will tell you that you can't treat a virus, because antibiotics don't work on viruses. But Oriental medicine and naturopathy take a different approach: rather than using a 'magic bullet' like an antibiotic, it works to strengthen the immune system so that your body fights the virus itself. The body naturally wants to heal itself, but sometimes you have to give it a little extra nudge.

This 'positive and preventive health' approach is all part of my philosophy of being kind to yourself. I really think it's important to keep your stress levels under control; to eat well and to give yourself plenty of TLC. And, for me, that includes working on achieving optimum health. Without it, I can't work. I can't sing! And I have to sing to stay happy...

Pure *Intuition*

Women are lucky: I think we're naturally more intuitive than men. So there is one very important voice in my life, apart from my singing voice — and that's my inner voice. Sometimes I can make snap judgements. But often I don't know the answer immediately so I will sit with an idea for a time, while I wait for my inner voice to tell me what to do. If you work on that inner stillness — especially through meditation — then I believe it's easier to tune into that intuition and make the choices that are right for you at that moment in time. Honestly, it can be something like 'Do I really *need* that pint of Häagen-Dazs that's calling my name from the freezer?' To which the answer is clearly, 'No!' So I just listen to my intuition — right through to career choices. Big decisions, little decisions. And I find that they are all easier when I create the stillness and silence that makes it easier for that inner voice to be heard...

'THIS "POSTIVE AND PREVENTIVE" HEALTH APPROACH IS ALL PART OF MY PHILOSOPHY OF BEING KIND TO YOURSELF.'

'If by strength is meant moral power, then woman is immeasurably man's superior. Has she not greater intuition, is she not more self-sacrificing, has she not greater power of endurance, has she not greater courage? Without her man could not be. If non-violence is the law of our being, the future is with woman. Who can make a more affective appeal to the heart than woman?'

Mahatma Gandhi

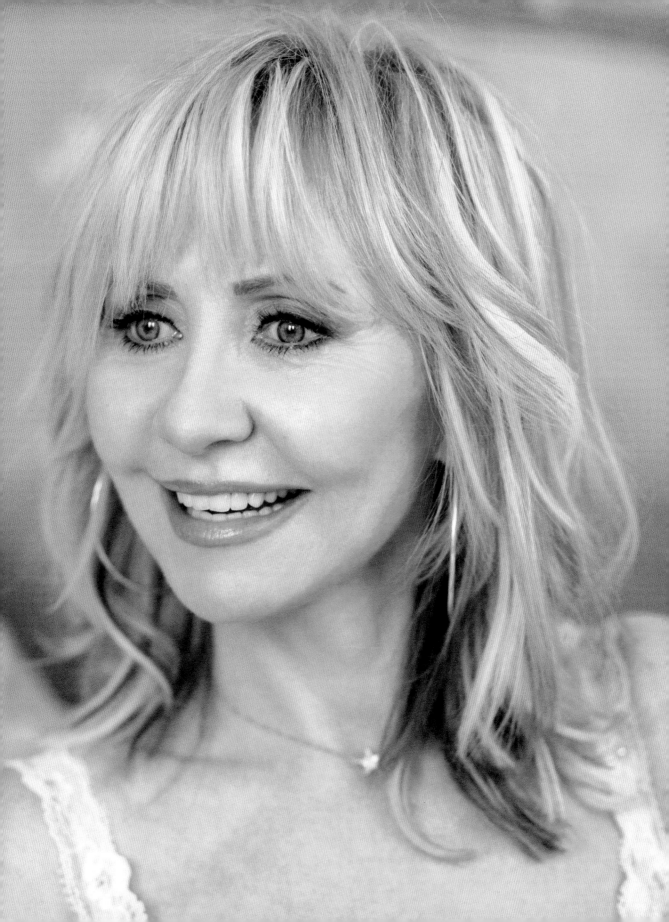

Feel The Music

Music and singing are my life. They are food for my soul, what makes me tick. It's almost a spiritual thing, to be honest. I hope that you have a passion in your life that does for you what music does for me — and, if not, then go out in this world and *find* it. I have my parents to thank for my love of popular music. They liked Sinatra and popular American music, bought hit records. I became interested in Ray Charles, The Drifters, Sam Cooke and Sister Rosetta Tharp being played in our house. My parents were obsessed with American music: for me, it was soul, R & B and rock music, with a large helping of gospel thrown in. There were a couple of air bases near Glasgow where I used to sing with my band, and I just loved hearing that American music on the jukebox. On Friday and Saturday nights the pubs would close and my parents' friends would often pile back to my parents' house for homemade food and whisky and singing. I'd bring my brother down and, standing in the middle of the room in my PJs, I'd put on impromptu concerts and wouldn't stop until my mum and dad literally pushed me out of the room to send me to bed...

Now, my mother would insist that I could sing before I could talk — which is ridiculous, but you know what? It's true. I think it all went back to the fact that my father used to walk around the house singing at the top of his voice. In Scotland, when babies were fractious, they were swaddled in shawls and kept close to their mother's or father's heart, and they'd 'shoogle' the baby up and down with the idea that the gentle movement and the heartbeat would soothe that anxiety. Well, my dad used to do that with me, but he'd also sing while he did it. He used to tell me that I'd actually press my ear to his cheek: I wanted to hear the vibration of his voice inside my head.

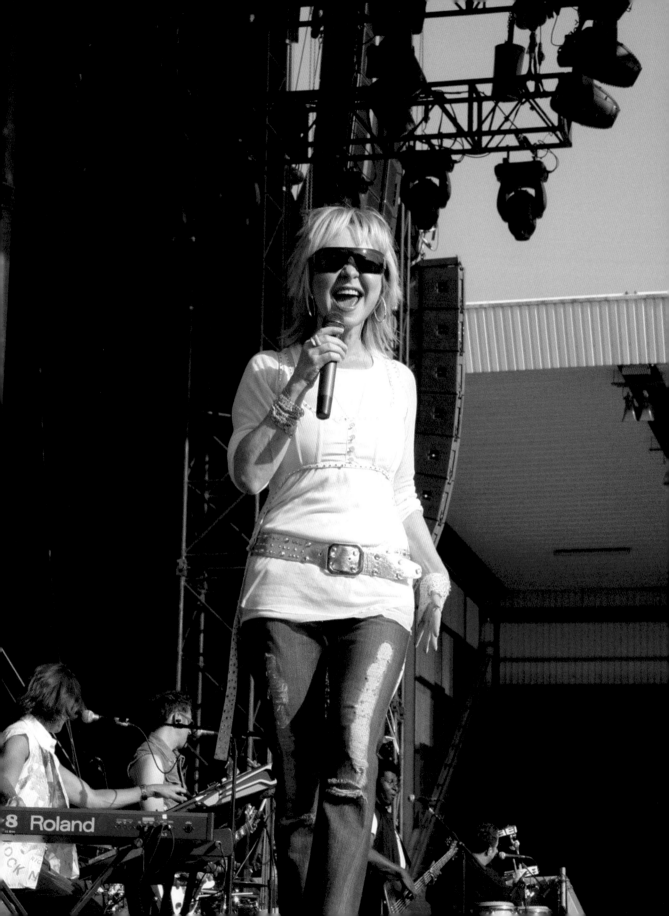

Do it *Now*

* *Sign up for that class you've always wanted to take…*

* *Go for a long walk and make sure that it's further than you've ever walked before…*

* *Change your lipstick…*

* *Make friends with younger people, not just those your own age…*

* *Take a dance class…*

* *Have that makeover in a department store you've been promising yourself…*

* *Challenge yourself, all the time…*

These are the true secrets of staying young…

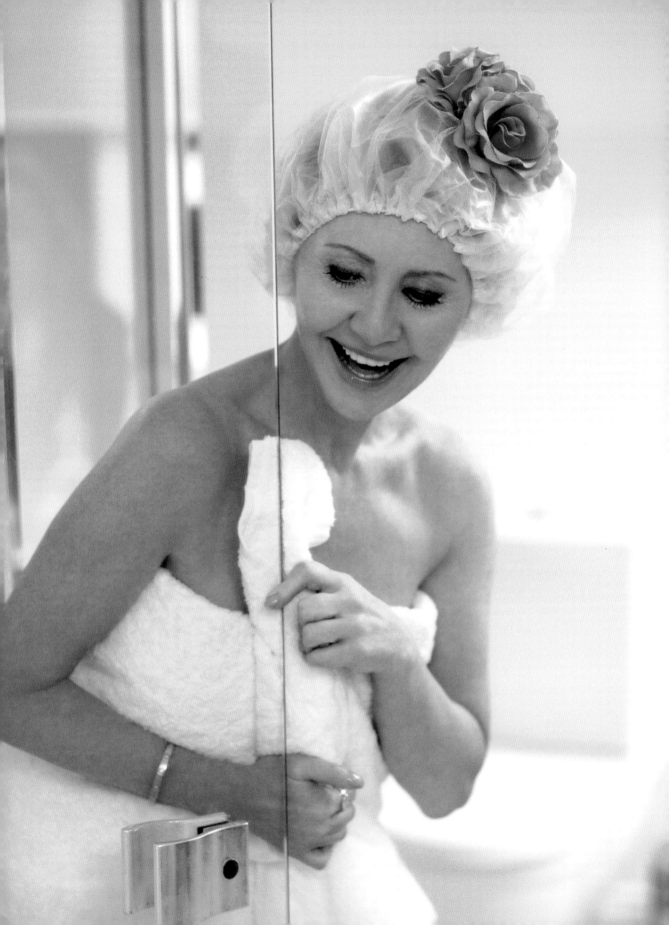

Lulu's *Golden* Rules

I live by these rules — and I hope you find them helpful, too...

✱ *Don't get stuck in a rut*

Experiment! Play with your hair, your make-up, your clothes, your accessories. One of the most ageing things in life is to be 'freeze-framed' with a particular style — or a particular mindset. Playing is youthful — it's what children do. So don't stop...

✱ *Give your skin plenty of TLC*

If your skin glows, that's the first thing everyone notices. The secret to radiance is exfoliation — it's dull, dead cells that look old, so buff them away daily. And that way your skin is prepared for everything you apply afterwards...

✱ *Work on your inner calm*

Life throws challenges at us all the time — but if you have an inner stillness and strength, you are better able to handle them. Try yoga and meditation, or find a formula that works for you, and every day spend a little time developing your inner strength.

✳ Stay flexible

I mean that literally! Yoga and pilates are both incredible for keeping you supple as well as strong, which has been shown to help prevent falls in later life. So s-t-r-e-t-c-h every single day.

✳ Remember, when it comes to make-up, less is more

Don't be tempted to use make-up like Polyfilla to cover up what you see as your flaws. Use a lighter touch after a certain age.

✳ Stay out of the sun

At the very least, keep your face out of the sun. Prevention is much, much easier than cure and sun damage is your skin's number-one worst enemy, so keep it protected as much as you possibly can.

✳ Get regular health checks

Better to be safe than sorry.

✳ Accentuate the positive

What are your best features — your hair, your slim wrists and ankles, your skin? Play them up. Draw attention to the parts of yourself that you're happiest with and, trust me, that's all anyone will notice.

✳ *Eat 'positively', too*

When you sit down for a meal, try to choose the food which is going to most benefit your skin and body — healthy choices that boost health from within. Don't think about what you *shouldn't* have — you'll only want it more — but by focusing on eating what's going to nourish you the best, it's easier to stay away from the junkier foods and drinks.

✳ *Have a glass of water before you eat*

It helps hydrate you and fills part of your stomach. (Much better than drinking *with* your meal which can interfere with your digestion.)

✳ *Don't be hard on yourself*

Nobody's perfect. If you have a biscuit binge one day, or realise you haven't exercised in a while, don't give up: get back to your good habits. Above all, be kind to yourself.

✳ *Enjoy every moment*

We are here for a very short time. Spend that time as positively as you can, enjoying every moment to its fullest potential — filling your life with music, colour, love. We all want to look fabulous, yes. But there's more to life. Cherish friends, family and colleagues and try to see the positive in everything. Because there is *always* a positive...

✳ *Laugh!*

It really is the best medicine of all... Because after a good belly laugh, you always, always feel better.

Directory

Skin

Arezoo
Beauty therapists
020 7584 6868
www.arezoo.co.uk

Boots
Sunglasses
0845 070 8090
www.boots.com

Cutler & Gross
Sunglasses
020 7581 2250
www.cutlerandgross.com

Lulu's Time Bomb
Skincare products
0844 800 1694
www.lulusplace.co.uk

Micheline Arcier Aromathérapie
Aromatherapy
020 7235 3545
www.michelinearcier.com

Neal's Yard Remedies
Essential oils and base oils
0845 262 3145
www.nealsyardremedies.com

Make-up

Many of the following brands are widely available in department stores, but can also be found online at the following sites:

Anya Hindmarch
Make-up bags
020 7501 0177
www.anyahindmarch.com

Bobbi Brown
Make-up
www.bobbibrown.co.uk

By Terry
Skincare and make-up range
020 8740 2085
www.spacenk.co.uk

Dior
Make-up
020 7216 0216
www.beauty.dior.com

Jay Strongwater
Beautiful make-up accessories
www.jaystrongwater.com

Jenny Jordan
Eyebrow and make-up clinic
22 Englands Lane
Belsize Park
London NW3 4TG
020 7483 2222
www.jennyjordan.co.uk

Lancôme
Make-up
www.lancome.co.uk
www.boots.com

Laura Mercier
Make-up and skincare
www.lauramercier.com
www.spacenk.com

M.A.C.
Make-up
0870 034 6700
www.maccosmetics.co.uk

Maybelline
Make-up
0845 399 0304
www.maybelline.co.uk

Myface Cosmetics
www.myfacecosmetics.com
0844 335 6492
(Also at selected Boots stores)

Scott Barnes
Make-up
www.scottbarnes.com
www.hqhair.com

Shu Uemura
Make-up and skincare
www.spacenk.co.uk

Stila
Make-up
www.hqhair.com
http://www.stilacosmetics.com

Hair

Accessorize
www.monsoon.co.uk/icat/accessorize

Connect
Hair extensions
5 Adelaide Tavern
Adelaide Road
London NW3 3QE
www.connecthairextensions.com

John Frieda
4 Aldford Street
London W1W 6XA
020 7491 0840
www.johnfrieda.com

75 New Cavendish Street
London W1G 7LT
020 7636 1401

Kirby Grips
Look for 'Triple wave grips'
www.salonsdirect.com

Mason-Pearson hairbrushes
020 7491 2613
www.masonpearson.com
www.HQhair.com

Velcro rollers
www.salonsdirect.com

Body

Anna Ashby
Yoga instructor
www.annaashby.com

Bridget Woods Kramer
Yoga instructor
www.omshop.com

Canyon Ranch
Resort and hotel
www.canyonranch.com

Dyna-Band
Equipment for resistance work
www.dynaband.co.uk
(0)845 3054131

Essie
Nail products
www.essie.com
www.nailsbymail.co.uk

Jonathan Goodair
Personal trainer
www.jonathangoodair.com

Olivina
Hand cream and products
www.olivinanapavalley.com

Food

Books by Gaylord Hauser and
Gloria Swanson
www.abebooks.com

Chocolate Vianesse Powder and
Protein powder
For Sin-Free Brownie recipe
www.gfcfshakes.co.uk

Clearspring
Organic and traditional foods
www.clearspring.co.uk

Green & Black's
Chocolate producer
www.greenandblacks.com

Judges Bakery
For Sourdough bread
www.judgesbakery.com

The River Café
Thames Wharf
Rainville Road
London
W6 9HA
020 7386 4200
www.rivercafe.co.uk

Weight Watchers
Weight-loss support
www.weightwatchers.co.uk

Xylitol
Planet Organic
For Xylitol or other health food products
020 7221 1345
www.planetorganic.com
Or shop online at:
www.healthy.co.uk

Clothes

Accessorize
See HAIR

Browns
www.brownsfashion.com

Butler & Wilson
www.butlerandwilson.co.uk

Converse All Stars
www.justconverse.co.uk

Christian Louboutin
www.matchesfashion.com

Fendi
www.fendi.com

Gap
www.gap.com

Goyard
www.goyard.com

Guerlain
www.debenhams.com

The Holding Company
www.theholdingcompany.co.uk

H&M
www.hm.com

Hanky Pankies
www.stylefinder.com

IKEA
www.ikea.co.uk

James Perse
www.jamesperse.com
In the UK, visit www.shopstyle.co.uk (this
useful site tells you which other websites
are carrying which elements of each
designer range)

Loree Rodkin
In the UK, visit www.shopstyle.co.uk (see
above, under James Perse)

Miss Selfridge
www.missselfridge.com

Primark
www.primark.co.uk

Rick Owens
In the UK, visit www.shopstyle.co.uk (see
above, under James Perse)

Rigby & Peller
www.rigbyandpeller.com

Swarovski
www.swarovski.com

Stella McCartney
www.stellamccartney.com

SUN (fake tans)
www.qvc.co.uk

The Alexander Technique
www.alexandertechnique.org.uk

Theory
In the UK, visit www.shopstyle.co.uk (see
above, under James Perse)

Topshop
www.topshop.com

Trinny and Susannah's Magic
Knickers
www.figleaves.com

Velvet
www.misamu.com

Wolford
www.tightsplease.co.uk

Zara
www.zara.com

On My Bookshelf...

A New Earth (Penguin)
Eckhart Tolle

Courage to Change: One Day at a Time in Al-Anon II,
(Al-Anon Family Headquarters Inc.)
Al-Anon Family Group

Dreams from my Father
(Canongate Books)
Barack Obama

I Can Do It: How to Use Affirmations to Change Your Life
(Hay House Inc.)
Louise Hay

The Power of Now
(Mobius)
Eckhart Tolle

The Road Less Travelled
(Rider & Co.)
M. Scott Peck

Three Cups of Tea
(Penguin)
Greg Mortenson

Where Are You Going?
(SYDA Foundation)
Swami Muktananda

All books above are available via www.amazon.co.uk and other high street bookshops

Picture Credits and Acknowledgements

Photographers

p.6, 12, 23, 32, 39, 40, 43, 44, 49, 50, 72, 80-1, 93, 104, 128-9, 134, 148-9, 156, 168-9, 176-7, 187, 193, 197 (Bottom Right), 203, 211, 215, 231, 232, 253, 258 © Paul Cox.

p.17 (Top Right), 21, 26, 29, 31, 36, 56, 69 (Top Right, Middle), 78, 162, 164, 171-3, 195, 197 (Top Left, Top Right), 199, 204, 209, 220, 222, 224, 226, 231, 242, 244, 248 © Noel Murphy.

pp.113-25, 139-46 © Jerry Young.

p.17 (Top Left), 69 (Top Left, Bottom Left, Bottom Right), 87, 97, 126-27, 131, 229, 255, 197 (Bottom Left), 229, 255 Lulu's own archive.

Stock Photography

p.15 (Harry Goodwin/Redferns), p.17 (Bottom Left), 46-7 (Larry Ellis/Express/Getty Images), p.17 (Bottom Right), 75 (Bettmann/Corbis), p.35 (Steve Wood/Express/Getty Images), p.59 (Tom Hanley/Redferns/musicpictures.com), p.62, 88-9 © Photoshot, p.65 (Simon James/WireImage/Getty Images), p.100 (Alamy), p.133 (Courtesy of EMI Archives), p.182-3, 218-19 (Michael Ochs Archives/Getty Images), p.184, 240 (Hulton-Deutsch Collection/Corbis).

Acknowledgement's go to my personal team.
In the overall creative direction of this project –
Gail Federici and Kim Livingston.
To Steven Howard my manager and all at TCB.
Jo Fairley – for putting my thoughts in to words so brilliantly.
My Glam Squad – Kevin Moss, Gemma Smith-Edhouse and Jillie Murphy.
Claire Finbow – Personal Assistant to Lulu.
A special thanks to Bonnie who brought me so much joy for 18 years and is now in doggy heaven.

The Publisher would like to thank the following people for their contribution to the book:
The team at TCB Management, Jo Fairley, photographers Paul Cox, Noel Murphy and Jerry Young, yoga instructor Anna Ashby and personal trainer Jon Goodair, stylists Jillie Murphy, Nel Haynes, Kimberley Watson and Tamsin Weston, designers Martin Topping and Jilly Sitford of 'Ome Design, Steve Crozier of Butterfly Creative Services.

Credits

p.159, 166, 167 'The River Café's Braised Swiss Chard with Chilli and Garlic' recipe, 'Salsa Rosso' recipe and 'Salsa Verde' recipe, taken from *The River Café Cook Book* by Rose Gray and Ruth Rogers, published by Ebury. Reprinted by permission of The Random House Group Ltd.

p.44 MAC lip pencil in Subculture, p.56 MAC eyeshadows, p.69 MAC Professional brushes, courtesy of MAC Cosmetics.

Index